Awareness
through
Movement

AWARENESS THROUGH MOVEMENT

Health Exercises for Personal Growth

MOSHE FELDENKRAIS

ILLUSTRATED EDITION

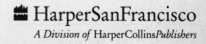
HarperSanFrancisco

A Division of HarperCollins*Publishers*

FIRST HARPERCOLLINS PAPERBACK EDITION PUBLISHED IN 1990.

Library of Congress Cataloging-in-Publication Data

Feldenkrais, Moshe
   Awareness through movement : health exercises for personal growth /
Moshe Feldenkrais. — 1st HarperCollins pbk. ed.
   p. cm.
   ISBN 0-06-250322-7
   1. Feldenkrais method.   I. Title.
RC489.F44F44   1990   90-55454
613.7—dc20

95 96 RRD 10 9 8 7 6

"Awareness Through Movement" has served as the introduction for thousands of people to the Feldenkrais Method. In my travels with Moshe Feldenkrais, and during the workshops he presented, people would come up and tell us how this book made a great difference in their lives — assisting them in recovering from great personal difficulties and enriching the quality of their lives.

Kolman Korentayer, a gestalt and Feldenkrais practitioner, was North America Co-ordinator of Feldenkrais Programs, 1970-1979.

Contents

PART ONE
Understanding While Doing

Preface

We act in accordance with our self-image. This self-image—which, in turn, governs our every act—is conditioned in varying degree by three factors: heritage, education, and self-education.

The part that is inherited is the most immutable. The biological endowment of the individual—the form and capacity of his nervous system, his bone structure, muscles, tissue, glands, skin, senses—are all determined by his physical heritage long before he has any established identity. His self-image develops from his actions and reactions in the normal course of experience.

Education determines one's language and establishes a pattern of concepts and reactions common to a specific society. These concepts and reactions will vary according to the environment into which a person is born; they are not characteristic of mankind as a species, but only of certain groups or individuals.

Education largely determines the direction of our self-education, which is the most active element in our development and in more frequent use socially than elements of biological origin. Our self-education influences the manner in which external education is acquired, as well as the selection of the material to be learned and the rejection of that which we cannot assimilate. Education and self-education occur intermittently. In the first weeks of an infant's life, education is chiefly a matter of absorbing the environment, and self-education is almost nonexistent; it consists only of refusal of, or resistance to, anything that is organically alien and unacceptable to the infant's inherited characteristics.

Self-education progresses as the infant organism grows and becomes more stable. The child gradually develops individual characteristics; he begins to choose among objects and actions in accordance with his own nature. He no longer accepts everything that training tries to impose on him. Imposed education and individual propensities together set the trend for all our habitual behavior and actions.

Of the three active factors in the establishment of our self-image, self-education alone is to some extent in our own hands. Our physical inheritance comes to us unsolicited, education is forced upon us, and even self-education is not entirely volitional in the early years; it is decided by the relative strength of inherited personality, individual characteristics, the effective working of the nervous system, and by the severity and persistence of educational influences. Heritage makes each one of us a unique individual in physical structure, appearance, and actions. Education makes each of us a member of some definite human society and seeks to make us as like every other member of that society as possible. Society dictates our mode of dress, and thereby makes our appearance similar to that of others. By giving us a language, it makes us express ourselves in the same way as others. It instills a pattern of behavior and values in us and sees to it that our self-education shall also operate so as to make us wish to become like everyone else.

As a result, even self-education, which is the active force that makes for individuality and extends inherited difference into the realm of action, tends to a large extent to bring our behavior into line with that of others. The essential flaw in education as we know it today is that it is based on ancient and often primitive practices whose equalizing purpose was neither conscious nor clear. This flaw has its advantage since, having no defined purpose other than to mold individuals who will not be social misfits, education does not always succeed entirely in suppressing self-education. Nonetheless, even in the advanced countries, in which educational methods are constantly improving, there is increasing similarity of opinions, appearance, and ambitions. The development of mass communication and political aspirations to equality also contribute significantly to the present heightened blurring of identities.

Modern knowledge and techniques in the fields of education and psychology have already enabled Professor B. F. Skinner, the Harvard psychologist, to demonstrate methods for the production of individuals who are "satisfied, capable, educated, happy, and creative." This is also, in effect, the aim of education, even though it is not expressly so stated. Skinner is certainly right about the effectiveness of these methods, and there is little doubt that in time we shall be able to develop units in the form of man that are educated, organized, satisfied, and happy; if we use all our knowledge in the field of biological inheritance, we may even succeed in producing several different types of such units to satisfy all the needs of society.

This utopia, which has a feasible chance of happening in our lifetime, is the logical outcome of the present situation. In order to bring it about we need only produce biological uniformity and employ suitable educational measures to prevent self-education.

Many people feel that the community is more important than the individuals of which it is composed. A trend toward the improvement of the community is found in almost all advanced countries, the difference being only in the methods chosen to realize this goal. There seems to be general agreement that the most important thing is to improve the social processes of employment, production, and provision of equal opportunities for all. In every society care is taken that the education of the younger generation should result in qualities making for as uniform a community as possible that will then function without any great disturbance.

It may be that these tendencies of society agree with the evolutionary trend of the human species; if so, everyone should certainly direct his efforts toward the achievement of this aim.

If, however, we for a moment disregard the concept of society and turn to man himself, we see that society is not merely the sum total of the people who constitute it; from the individual's point of view it has a different meaning. It has import for him, first of all, as the field in which he must advance in order to be accepted as a valuable member, his value in his own eyes being influenced by his position in society. It is also important to him as a field in which he may exercise his individual qualities, develop and give expression to particular personal inclinations that are organic to his personality. Organic traits derive from his biological inheritance, and their expression is essential for the maximal functioning of the organism. As the trend to uniformity within our society creates innumerable conflicts with individual traits, adjustments to society can be solved either by the suppression of the individual's organic needs, or by the individual's identification with the society's needs (in a manner that does not appear to him to be imposed), which may go so far as to make the individual feel that he is debased whenever he fails to behave in accordance with society's values.

The education provided by society operates in two directions at once. It suppresses every noncomformist tendency through penalties of withdrawal of support and simultaneously imbues the individual with values that force him to overcome and discard spontaneous desires. These conditions cause the majority of adults today to live behind a mask, a mask of personality that the individual tries to present to others and to himself. Every aspiration and spontaneous desire is subjected to stringent internal criticism lest they reveal the individual's organic nature. Such aspirations and desires arouse anxiety and remorse and the individual seeks to suppress the urge to realize them. The only compensation that makes life durable despite these sacrifices is the satisfaction derived from society's recognition of the individual who achieves its definition of success. The need for constant support by one's fellows is so great that most people spend the larger part of their lives fortifying their masks. Repeated success is essential to encourage the individual to persist in this masquerade.

This success must be visible, involving a constant climb up the socioeconomic ladder. If he fails in the climb, not only will his living conditions become more difficult, but his value will diminish in his own eyes to the point of endangering his mental and physical health. He can scarcely allow himself time for a vacation, even if he has the material means. The actions and the drive that produces them—necessary in order to maintain a mask free of flaws and cracks lest he be revealed behind it—do not derive from any basic organic needs. As a result, the satisfaction derived from these actions even when they are successful is not a revitalizing organic satisfaction, but merely a superficial, external one.

Very slowly, over the years, a man comes to convince himself that society's recognition of his success should and does give him organic contentment. Often enough the individual becomes so adjusted to his mask, his identification with it so complete, that he no longer senses any organic drive or satisfactions. This can result in the revelation of flaws and disturbances in family and sex relations that may always have been present but that have been glossed over by the individual's success in society. And, indeed, the private organic life and the gratification of needs deriving from strong organic drives are almost unimportant to the successful existence of the mask and to its social value. The great majority of people live active and satisfactory enough lives behind their masks to enable them to stifle more or less painlessly any emptiness they may feel whenever they stop and listen to their heart.

Not everyone succeeds in occupations that society considers important to the degree that enables them to live a satisfactory mask-life. Many of those who fail in their youth to acquire a profession or trade that would offer them sufficient prestige to maintain their mask-lives claim that they are lazy and have neither the character nor the persistence to learn anything. They try their hand at one thing after another, switch from job to job, invariably considering themselves nonetheless fit for whatever may turn up next. This confidence in their own abilities gives them sufficient organic satisfaction to make each stab at something new worth the effort. These people may be no less gifted than others, maybe even more so, but they have acquired the habit of disregarding their organic needs until they can no longer find genuine interest in any activity. They may happen to stumble upon something at which they may last longer than usual and even attain a certain proficiency. But it will still be chance that has given them an occupation and thereby a foothold in society that will justify their own assessment of their worth. At the same time their precarious self-regard will drive them to seek success in other spheres, as likely as not in promiscuous sex. This promiscuity, which parallels their constant changing of jobs, is activated by the same mechanism of belief in some special gift of their own. It raises their value in their own eyes and, again, gives them at least partial organic satisfaction; enough, in any event, to make it worth their while to try again.

Self-education—which, as we have seen, is not altogether independent—also causes other structural and functional conflicts. Thus, many people suffer some form of disturbance in digestion, elimination, breathing, or bone structure. Periodic improvements in one of these malfunctions will bring about improvement in the others, and increase general vitality for a time, followed in almost every instance by a period of lowered health and spirits.

It is obvious that of the three factors determining a man's general behavior, self-education alone is appreciably subject to will. The question is really to what extent and, most particularly, in what way one can help oneself. Most people will choose to consult an expert—the best answer in serious cases. However, most people do not recognize the need, nor have they any wish to do so; in any case, it is doubtful whether the expert will be of much use. Self-help is, in the final instance, the only way open to everyone.

This way is hard and complicated, but for every person who feels the need for change and improvement it is within the limits of practical possibility, bearing in mind that several things must be clearly understood to make the process, the acquisition of a new set of responses, not too difficult.

It must be fully realized from the start that the learning process is irregular and consists of steps, and that there will be downs as well as ups. This applies even to a matter as simple as learning a poem by heart.

A man may learn a poem one day, and remember almost nothing of it the next. A few days later, and without any further study, he may suddenly know it perfectly. Even if he puts the poem entirely out of his mind for several months, he will find that a brief rehearsal will bring it back completely. We must not become discouraged, therefore, if we find we have slipped back to the original condition at any time; these regressions will become rarer and return to the improved condition easier as the learning process continues.

It should further be realized that as changes take place in the self, new and hitherto unrecognized difficulties will be discovered. The consciousness previously rejected them either from fear or because of pain, and it is only as self-confidence increases that it becomes possible to identify them.

Most people make sporadic attempts to improve and correct themselves even though they are often done without any clear awareness of it. The average person is satisfied with his achievements and thinks he needs nothing except some gymnastics to correct a few acknowledged faults. Everything that has been said in this introduction is in fact addressed to this average man; that is, to the man who thinks none of it concerns him.

As people try to better themselves, different stages of development can be found in each of them. And as each one progresses, the means for further correction will have to become increasingly finespun. I have outlined in this book the first steps on this road in considerable detail to enable readers to go even further under their own power.

The
Self-Image

The dynamics of personal action

Each one of us speaks, moves, thinks, and feels in a different way, each according to the image of himself that he has built up over the years. In order to change our mode of action we must change the image of ourselves that we carry within us. What is involved here, of course, is a change in the dynamics of our reactions, and not the mere replacing of one action by another. Such a change involves not only a change in our self-image, but a change in the nature of our motivations, and the mobilization of all the parts of the body concerned.

These changes produce the noticeable difference in the way each individual carries out similar actions—handwriting and pronunciation, for instance.

The four components of action

Our self-image consists of four components that are involved in every action: movement, sensation, feeling, and thought. The contribution of each of the components to any particular action varies, just as the persons carrying out the action vary, but each component will be present to some extent in any action.

In order to think, for instance, a person must be awake, and know that he is awake and not dreaming; that is, he must sense and discern his physical position relative to the field of gravity. It follows that movement, sensing, and feeling are also involved in thinking.

In order to feel angry or happy, a man must be in a certain posture, and in some kind of relationship to another being or object. That is, he must also move, sense, and think.

In order to sense—see, hear, or touch—a person must be interested, startled, or aware of some happening that involves him. That is, he must move, feel, and think.

In order to move, he must use at least one of his senses, consciously or unconsciously, which involves feeling and thinking.

When one of these elements of action becomes so minute as almost to disappear, existence itself may be endangered. It is difficult to survive for even brief periods without any movement at all. There is no life where a being is deprived of all senses. Without feeling, there is no drive to live; it is the feeling of suffocation that forces us to breathe. Without at least some minimum of reflex thought, even a beetle cannot live too long.

Changes become fixed as habits

In reality our self-image is never static. It changes from action to action, but these changes gradually become habits; that is, the actions take on a fixed, unchanging character.

Early in life, when the image is being established, the rate of change in the image is high; new forms of action that had only the previous day been beyond the child's capacity are quickly achieved. The infant begins to see, for instance, a few weeks after birth; one day he will begin to stand, walk, and talk. The child's own experiences, together with his biological inheritance, combine slowly to create an individual way of standing, walking, speaking, feeling, listening, and of carrying out all the other actions that give substance to human life. But while from a distance the life of one person appears to be very similar to that of any other, on close inspection they are entirely different. We must, then, use words and concepts in such a way that they will apply more or less equally to everyone.

How the self-image is formed

We confine ourselves therefore to examining in detail the motor part of the self-image. Instinct, feeling, and thought being linked with movement, their role in the creation of the self-image reveals itself together with that of movement.

The stimulation of certain cells in the motor cortex of the brain will activate a particular muscle. It is known today that the correspondence between the cells of the cortex and the muscles that they activate is neither absolute nor exclusive. Nevertheless, we may consider that there is sufficient experimental justification to assume that specific cells do activate specific muscles at least in basic, elementary movements.

Individual and social action

The newborn human can perform practically nothing of what he will carry out as an adult in human society, but he can do almost everything the adult can do as an individual. He can breathe, eat, digest, eliminate, and his body can organize all the biological and physiological processes except the sexual act—and this may be considered a social process in the adult, for it takes place between two persons. In the beginning, sexual activity remains confined to the individual sphere. It is now widely accepted that adult sexuality develops from early self-sexuality. This approach makes it possible to explain inadequacies in this field as a failure in the development of the individual toward full social sexuality.

Contact with the external world

The infant's contact with the external world is established mainly through the lips and mouth; through these he recognizes his mother. He will use his hands to fumble and assist the work of his mouth and lips, and will know by touch what he already knows through his lips and mouth. From here he will gradually progress to the discovery of other parts of his body and their relationship to each other, and through them his first notions of distance and volume. The discovery of time begins with the coordinating of processes of breathing and swallowing, both of which are connected with movements of the lips, mouth, jaw, nostrils, and the surrounding area.

The self-image on the motor cortex

Were we to mark in color on the surface area of the motor cortex of the brain of a month-old infant the cells that activate muscles subject to his developing will, we should obtain a form resembling that of his body, but it would represent only the areas of voluntary action, not the anatomical configuration of the parts of his body. We should see, for instance, that the lips and mouth occupy most of the colored area. The antigravity muscles—those that open the joints and so erect the body —are not yet subject to voluntary control; the muscles of the hands, too, are only just beginning to respond occasionally to will. We should obtain a functional image in which the human body is indicated by four thin strokes of the pen for the limbs, joined together by another short and thin line for the trunk, with lips and mouth occupying most of the picture.

Every new function changes the image

Were we to color the cells activating muscles subject to voluntary control of a child that has already learned to walk and write, we should obtain quite a different functional image. The lips and mouth would again occupy most of the space because the function of speech, which involves the tongue, mouth, and lips, has been added to the previous picture. However another large patch of color would have become conspicuous, covering the area of cells that activate the thumbs. The area of cells activating the right thumb will be noticeably larger than that activating the left one. The thumb takes part in almost every movement made by the hand, in writing particularly. The area representing the thumb will be larger than that representing the other fingers.

The muscle-image in the motor cortex is unique for every individual

If we continued to draw such outlines every few years, not only would the result be different each time, but it would vary distinctively from one individual to another. In a man who has not learned to write, the patches of color representing the thumbs would remain small, because cells that might have been included would remain unused. The area for the third finger would be larger in a person who has learned to play a musical instrument than in one who has not. People who know several languages, or who sing, would show larger areas covering cells that activate the muscles for the control of breathing, tongue, mouth, and so on.

Only the muscle-image is based on observation

In the course of much experimenting, physiologists have discovered that in basic movements at least, the cells concerned link up on the motor cortex of the brain into a shape resembling the body, which they refer to as the *homunculus*. There is thus a valid basis for the concept of the "self-image," at least in so far as basic movements are concerned. We have no similar experimental evidence with regard to sensation, feeling, or thought.

Our self-image is smaller than our potential capacity

Our self-image is essentially smaller than it might be, for it is built up only of the group of cells that we have actually used. Further, the various patterns and combinations of cells are perhaps more important than their actual number. A man who has mastered several languages will make use both of more cells and more combinations of cells. Most children of minority population communities the world over know at least two languages; their self-image is a little nearer the potential maximum than that of people who know only their mother tongue.

It is the same in most other areas of activity. Our self-image is in general more limited and smaller than our potential. There are individuals who know from thirty to seventy languages. This indicates that the average self-image occupies only about 5 percent of its potential. Systematic observation and treatment of some thousands of individuals drawn from most nations and civilizations have convinced me that this figure is roughly the fraction we use of our total hidden potential.

The achievement of immediate objectives has a negative aspect

The negative aspect of learning to achieve aims is that we tend to stop learning when we have mastered sufficient skills to attain our immediate objective. Thus, for instance, we improve our speech until we can make ourselves understood. But any person who wishes to speak with the clarity of an actor discovers that he must study speech for several years in order to achieve anything approaching his maximum potential in this direction. An intricate process of limiting ability accustoms man to make do with 5 percent of his potential without realizing that his development has been stunted. The complexity of the situation is brought about by the inherent interdependence between the growth and development of

the individual and the culture and economy of the society in which he
grows.

Education is largely tied to prevailing circumstances

Nobody knows the purpose of life, and the education that each
generation passes on to the succeeding one is no more than a continuation of the habits of thought of the prevailing generation. Life has been
a harsh struggle since the beginning of mankind; nature is not kind to
creatures lacking awareness. One cannot ignore the great social difficulties created by the existence of the many millions of people the earth
has harbored in the past few centuries. Under such conditons of strain,
education is improved only to the extent that is necessary and possible
in order to bring up a new generation able to replace the old one under
more or less similar conditions.

Minimum development of the individual satisfies the needs of society

The basic biological tendency of any organism to grow and develop
to its fullest extent has been largely governed by social and economic
revolutions that improved living conditions for the majority and enabled
greater numbers to reach a minimum of development. Under these
conditions basic potential development ceased in early adolescence because the demands of society enabled the members of the young generation to be accepted as useful individuals at the minimum stage. Further
training after early adolescence is, in fact, confined to the acquisition of
practical and professional knowledge in some field, and basic development is continued only by chance and in exceptional cases. Only the
unusual person will continue to improve his self-image until it more
nearly approaches the potential ability inherent in each individual.

The vicious circle of incomplete development and satisfaction with achievement

In the light of the statements above, it becomes clear that most people do not achieve the use of more than a minute fraction of their potential ability; the minority that outstrips the majority does so not because of its higher potential, but because it learns to use a higher proportion of this potential, that may well be no more than average—taking into account of course that no two people share an identical natural ability.

How is such a vicious circle created, which at one and the same time stunts men's powers, yet permits them to feel reasonably self-satisfied for all that they have limited themselves to, a small proportion of their capacities? It is a curious situation.

The physiological processes that hamper development

In the first years of his life, man is similar to every other living being, mobilizing all his separate powers and using every function that is sufficiently developed. The cells of his body seek, like all living cells, to grow and to perform their specific functions. This applies equally to the cells of the nervous system; each one lives its own life as a cell while participating in the organic function for which it exists. Nevertheless many cells remain inactive as part of the total organism. This may be because of two different processes. In one, the organism may be occupied with actions that require the inhibition of certain cells and the necessary mobilization of others. If the body is occupied more or less continuously with such actions, then a number of cells will be in an almost constant state of inhibition.

In the other case, some potential functions may not reach maturity at all. The organism may have no call to practice them, either because it sets no value on them as such, or because its drives lead it in a different direction. Both these processes are common. And, indeed, social conditions allow an organism to function as a useful member of society without in the least developing its capacities to the full.

Man judges himself in accordance with his value to society

The general tendency toward social improvement in our day has led directly to a disregard, rising to neglect, for the human material of which society is built. The fault lies not in the goal itself—which is constructive in the main—but in the fact that individuals, rightly or wrongly, tend to identify their self-images with their value to society. Even if he has emancipated himself from his educators and protectors, man does not strive to make himself any different from the pattern impressed upon him from the outset. In this way society comes to be made up of persons increasingly alike in their ways, behavior, and aims. Despite the fact that the inherited differences between people are obvious, there are few individuals who view themselves without reference to the value attributed to them by society. Like a man trying to force a square peg into a round hole, so the individual tries to smooth out his biological peculiarities by alienating himself from his inherent needs. He strains to fit himself into the round hole that he now actively desires to fill, for if he fails in this, his value will be so diminished in his own eyes as to discourage further initiative. These considerations must be borne in mind to appreciate fully the overwhelming influence of the individual's attitude toward himself once he again seeks to foster his own growth, that is, to allow his specific qualities to develop and reach fruition.

Judging a child by his achievements robs him of spontaneity

During his early years a child is valued, by and large, not for his achievements, but simply for himself. In families where this is the case, the child will develop in accordance with his individual abilities. In families where children are judged primarily by their achievements, all spontaneity will disappear at an early age. These children will become adults without experiencing adolescence. Such adults may from time to time feel an unconscious longing for the adolescence they have missed, a desire to seek out those instinctive capacities within themselves that were denied their youthful will to develop.

Self-improvement is linked to recognition of the value of the self

It is important to understand that if a man wishes to improve his self-image, he must first of all learn to value himself as an individual, even if his faults as a member of society appear to him to outweigh his qualities.

We may learn from persons crippled from birth or childhood how an individual may view himself in the face of obvious shortcomings. Those who succeed in looking at themselves with a sufficient, encompassing humanity to achieve stable self-respect may reach heights that the normally healthy will never achieve. But those who consider themselves inferior because of their disabilities, and overcome them by sheer will power, tend to grow into hard and embittered adults who will take revenge upon fellow men who are not at fault and, moreover, who may not be able to change the circumstances even if they wished to do so.

Action becomes the main arm in furthering self-improvement

Recognizing one's value is important at the start of self-improvement, but for any real improvement to be achieved, regard for the self will have to be relegated to second place. Unless a stage is reached at which self-regard ceases to be the main motivating force, any improvement achieved will never be sufficient to satisfy the individual. In fact, as a man grows and improves, his entire existence centers increasingly on *what* he does and how, while *who* does it becomes of ever decreasing importance.

The difficulty of changing an earlier pattern of action

A man tends to regard his self-image as something bestowed upon him by nature, although it is, in fact, the result of his own experience. His appearance, voice, way of thinking, environment, his relationship to space and time—to choose at random—are all taken for granted as realities born with him, whereas every important element in the individual's relationship to other people and to society in general is the result of extensive training. The arts of walking, speaking, reading, and of recognizing three dimensions in a photograph are skills the individual accumulates over a period of many years; each of them depends on chance, and on the place and period of his birth. The acquisition of a second language is not as easy as that of the first, and the pronunciation of the newly learned language will be marked by the influence of the first; the sentence structure of the first language will impose itself on the second. Every pattern of action that has become fully assimilated will interfere with the patterns of subsequent actions.

Difficulties arise, for instance, when a person learns to sit according to the custom of some nation other than his own. As these early patterns of sitting are not the result of heredity alone, but derive from the chance and circumstances of birth, the difficulties involved lie less in the nature of the new habit than in the changing of habits of body, feeling, and mind from their established patterns. This holds true for almost any change of habit, whatever its origin. What is meant here, of course, is not the simple substitution of one activity by another, but a change in the way an act is performed, a change in its whole dynamics, so that the new method will be in every respect as good as the old.

There is no awareness of many parts of the body

A person who lies down on his back and tries to sense his entire body systematically—that is, turning his attention to every limb and part of the body in turn—finds that certain sections respond easily, while others remain mute or dull and beyond the range of his awareness.

It is thus easy to sense the fingertips or lips, but much harder to sense the back of the head at the nape, between the ears. Naturally, the degree of difficulty is individual, depending on the form of the self-image. Generally speaking, it will be difficult to find a person whose whole body is equally accessible to his awareness. The parts of the body that are easily defined in the awareness are those that serve man daily, while the parts that are dull or mute in his awareness play only an indirect role in his life and are almost missing from his self-image when he is in action.

A person who cannot sing at all cannot feel this function in his self-image except by an effort of intellectual extrapolation. He is not aware of any vital connection between the hollow space in his mouth and his ears or his breathing, as does the singer. A man who cannot jump will not be aware of those parts of the body involved that are clearly defined to a man who is able to jump.

A complete self-image is a rare and ideal state

A complete self-image would involve full awareness of all the joints in the skeletal structure as well as of the entire surface of the body— at the back, the sides, between the legs, and so on; this is an ideal condition and hence a rare one. We can all demonstrate to ourselves that everything we do is in accordance with the limits of our self-image and that this image is no more than a narrow sector of the ideal image. It is also easily observed that the relationship between different parts of the self-image changes from activity to activity and from position to position. This is not so easily seen under common conditions, owing to their very familiarity, but it is sufficient to imagine the body poised for an unfamiliar movement in order to realize that the legs, for instance, will appear to change in length, thickness, and other aspects from movement to movement.

Estimation of size varies in different limbs

If we try, for instance, to indicate the length of our mouth, with eyes closed, by means of the thumb and first finger of the right hand, and with both hands using the first finger of each, we shall obtain two different values. Not only will neither measurement correspond to the actual length of the mouth, but both may be several times too large or too small. Again, if we try, with eyes closed, to estimate the thickness of our chest by placing our hands this distance apart, horizontally and vertically, we are likely to get two quite different values, neither of which need be anywhere near the truth.

Close your eyes and stretch out your arms in front of you, about the width of the shoulders apart, and then imagine the point at which the ray of light traveling from the index finger of the right hand to the left eye will cross the ray of light traveling from the index finger of the left hand to the right eye. Now try to mark this crossing point using the thumb and index finger of the right hand; it is unlikely that the place chosen will seem correct when you open your eyes to look.

There are few people whose self-image is sufficiently complete for them to be able to identify the correct spot in this way. What is more, if the experiment is repeated using the thumb and index finger of the left hand, a different location will most likely be chosen for the same point.

The average approximation is far from the best that can be achieved

It is easy to show by means of unfamiliar movements that our self-image is in general far from the degree of completeness and accuracy that we ascribe to it. Our image is formed through familiar actions in which approximation to reality is improved by bringing into play several of the senses that tend to correct each other. Thus, our image is more accurate in the region in front of our eyes than behind us or above our heads, and in familiar positions such as sitting or standing.

If the difference between imagined values or positions—one estimated with eyes closed and one with eyes open—is not more than 20 or 30 percent, accuracy may be considered average, though not satisfactory.

Individuals act in accordance with their subjective image

The difference between image and reality may be as much as 300 percent and even more. Persons who normally hold their chests in a position as though air had been expelled by the lungs in an exaggerated fashion, with their chest both flatter than it should be and too flat to serve them efficiently, are likely to indicate its depth as several times larger than it is if asked to do so with their eyes closed. That is, the excessive flatness appears right to them, because any thickening of the chest appears to them a demonstrably exaggerated effort to expand their lungs. Normal expansion feels to them as a deliberately blown up chest would to another person.

The way a man holds his shoulders, head, and stomach; his voice and expression; his stability and manner of presenting himself—all are based on his self-image. But this image may be cut down or blown up to fit the mask by which its owner would like to be judged by his peers. Only the man himself can know which part of his outward appearance is fictitious and which is genuine. However, not everybody is capable of identifying himself easily, and one may be greatly helped by the experience of others.

Systematic correction of the image is more useful than correction of single actions

From what has been said about the self-image, it emerges that systematic correction of the image will be a quicker and more efficient approach than the correction of single actions and errors in modes of behavior, the incidence of which increases as we come to deal with smaller errors.

The establishment of an initial more or less complete, although approximate, image will make it possible to improve the general dynamics instead of dealing with individual actions piecemeal. This improvement may be likened to correcting playing on an instrument that is not properly tuned. Improving the general dynamics of the image becomes the equivalent of tuning the piano itself, as it is much easier to play correctly on an instrument that is in tune than on one that is not.

Strata of Development

The first stage: The natural way

In all human activity, it is possible to isolate three successive stages of development. Children speak, walk, fight, dance, and then rest. Prehistoric man also spoke, walked, ran, fought, danced, and rested. At first these things were done "naturally," that is, in the same way that animals perform whatever is necessary for their lives. Although these things come to us naturally they are by no means simple. Even the simplest human activity is no less a mystery than the pigeon's return home over great distances or the bee's construction of a hive.

The natural activities are a common heritage

All these natural activities function similarly in every person, just as they are similar among pigeons and among bees.

There are tribes in all parts of the world, even in isolated families on islands, who have learned to speak naturally, as well as to run, jump, fight, wear clothes, swim, dance, sew, weave wool, tan hides, make baskets, and so on. But in some places the natural activities have devel-

oped and branched out; in others they have remained unchanged from
earliest times.

Stage two is individual

At the times and places where there was new development we always find a special, individual stage. That is, certain persons found
their own personal, special way of carrying out the activities that
came naturally. One person may have found his own special way of
expressing himself, another a special way of running, a different way
of weaving or making baskets, or some other individual way of doing
something that was different from the natural way. When this personal method proved to have vital advantages, it tended to be
adopted by others. In this way the Australians acquired the art of
throwing boomerangs, the Swiss learned to yodel, the Japanese to
use judo, and the South Sea Islanders to use the crawl stroke in
swimming. This is the second stage.

Stage three: method and profession

When a certain process can be done in a number of ways, some-
body may appear who will see the importance in the process itself,
apart from the way it is carried out by any individual. He will find
something in common in individual performances and will define the
process as such. In this, the third stage, the process is being carried
out according to a specific method as the result of knowledge, and
no longer naturally.

If we study the history of the various trades practiced in the civi-
lized world, we can find these three stages in them almost without
exception. In the dawn of humanity people produced wonderful
drawings naturally. Leonardo da Vinci employed elementary princi-
ples of perspective, but it was only in the nineteenth century that
these were fully defined (by Monge); since then they have been
taught at every school of art.

The learned method ousts natural practices

We may observe how natural practices have gradually given way to acquired methods, to "professional" methods, and that society in general refuses to allow the individual the right to employ the natural method, forcing him instead to learn the accepted way before it will permit him to work.

The birth of a child, for instance, was once a natural process and women knew how to help one another in the hour of need. But when midwifery became an accepted method and the midwife had a diploma, the ordinary woman was no longer entitled or able to help another during a birth.

Today we can see the continued process of the development of consciously constructed systems in place of individual, intuitive methods, and how actions that were once carried out naturally are becoming professions reserved for specialists. Only a hundred years ago one could deal with the insane in the natural way. The management of a household is becoming a profession, and its furnishing has become the business of interior decorators. The same thing has happened in many other areas of activity, including mathematics, singing, acting, war, planning, thinking, and similar fields; they began as natural actions and continued through individual improvements to become systems and professions.

The simpler an action the more retarded is its development

Observation and study indicate that the simpler and more common an action is in the natural way, the longer delayed will be the third systematic stage. Accepted methods were developed for the weaving of carpets, for geometry, philosophy, and mathematics thousands of years ago. Walking, standing, and other basic activities are only now reaching the third, or systematic, stage.

In the course of his life every person passes through all three stages

in some of his activities; in many others he passes through only one stage
or through the first two. Every man is born into a definite period and
grows into a society where he finds different activities in various stages
of development: some in the first stage, some in the second, some in the
third.

The stages are difficult to define

Every man adjusts himself to his time. In certain actions the natural
way will be the limit of his achievements as well as the limit of society's
achievement; in other actions he will be expected to reach the second
stage and in many the third. This adjustment has obvious difficulties
because of the vagueness of the process. In many cases it is hard to tell
whether we should rely on the natural way or start from the beginning
and study the methodical stages.

Thus many people who are unable to either sing or dance explain this
by saying that they never learned how. But there are also many who sing
and dance naturally, and they are certain that no trained singers and
dancers know more than they do unless they are naturally more gifted.
There are many people who do not know how to play drums, do a high
or broad jump, play a flute, draw or solve puzzles, or do many other
activities that were never learned in any but the natural way in earlier
times; today they dare not even try to learn these arts by themselves
because recognized methods exist.

The power of the system is so great in their eyes that even the little
they learned in their childhood of these things is gradually expunged
from their self-image because they are occupied mainly with activities
that they learned systematically and consciously. While such people are
very useful to society, they lack spontaneity and their lives are difficult
in areas outside their professional, learned field.

We thus come back to the need to examine and improve our self-
image so that we can live in accordance with our natural constitution
and gifts and not in accordance with the self-image that was established
by chance, more or less without our knowledge.

Possible problems with the third stage

The systematic stage of action is not wholly advantageous. Its main disadvantage is that many people do not even try to do specialized things, and as a result never attempt the first two stages at all, which are within everyone's capacity. Nevertheless, the systematic stage is of great importance. It enables us to find ways of behaving and acting that are in accordance with our personal and inner needs, ways that we might not discover naturally, because circumstances and outside influences may have led us in other directions in which continued progress is impossible. Systematic study and awareness should provide man with a means of scanning all fields of action so he can find a place for himself where he can act and breathe freely.

Where to Begin and How

Methods for human correction

The problem of human correction—either through others or by one's own efforts—has preoccupied man throughout his history. Many systems were devised for this purpose: The various religions have tried to describe ways of behavior intended to bring about man's improvement. Different systems of analysis are intended to assist man to free himself from deep-seated compulsions in his behavior. "Esoteric"—that is, "internal"—systems practiced in Tibet, India, and Japan, and used in all periods of human history, have also influenced Judaism. The cabalists, Hassidim, and the less-known practitioners of "Mussar" (moralists) were more influenced by Zen and Raja Yoga than appears at first sight.

A whole series of methods of suggestion and hypnosis (whether of many people or of a single person) are also common today. At least fifty such methods are known to be used in different corners of the world that are considered to be *the* method by those who practice them.

States of human existence

Two states of existence are commonly distinguished: waking and sleeping. We shall define a third state: awareness. In this state the individual knows exactly what he is doing while awake, just as we sometimes know when awake what we dreamed while asleep. For instance, at forty a man may become aware that one of his legs is shorter than the other, only after having suffered backaches, having had X rays taken and the trouble diagnosed by a doctor. This is possible because the waking state in general more resembles sleep than awareness.

Sleep has always been considered a convenient state in which to induce improvement in man. Coué used the moments when an individual is just falling asleep for autosuggestion and sleep itself for suggestion. In hypnosis the subject is put into a state of partial or deep sleep in order to make him more amenable to suggestion. In certain modern methods sleep is used to teach mathematics or languages as well as for suggestion.

The waking state seems to be a good condition in which to learn processes that involve repetition and explanation, but not suggestion. Habits acquired in the waking state are difficult to change, but they present little hindrance in grasping new matter.

The components of the waking state

Four components make up the waking state: sensation, feeling, thought, and movement. Each one serves as a basis for a whole series of methods of correction.

In *sensation* we include, in addition to the five familiar senses, the kinesthetic sense, which comprises pain, orientation in space, the passage of time, and rhythm.

In *feeling* we include—apart from the familiar emotions of joy, grief, anger, and so forth—self-respect, inferiority, supersensitivity, and other conscious and unconscious emotions that color our lives.

Thinking includes all functions of intellect, such as the opposition of right and left, good and bad, right and wrong; understanding, knowing that one understands, classifying things, recognizing rules, imagining, knowing what is sensed and felt, remembering all the above, and so on.

Movement includes all temporal and spatial changes in the state and configurations of the body and its parts, such as breathing, eating, speaking, blood circulation, and digestion.

Talking about separate components is an abstraction

The exclusion of any one of the four components is justified only in speech; in reality, not a moment passes in the waking state in which all man's capacities are not employed together. It is impossible, for instance, for you to recall an event, person, or landscape without using at least one of the senses—sight, hearing, or taste—to recapture the memory together with your self-image at the time, such as your position, your age, appearance, action, or pleasant or unpleasant feelings.

It follows from this interaction that detailed attention to any of these components will influence the others, hence the whole person. In reality there is no practical way of correcting an individual except by gradual improvement, alternating between the whole and its parts.

Differences in systems seem greater in theory than in practice

The real differences between the various correction systems is not so much in what they do as in what they say they do. Explicitly or implicitly, most of the systems are built on the assumption that man has innate propensities that can be changed—that is, suppressed, controlled, or inhibited. All systems that maintain that man has a fixed character consider each of his qualities, properties, and gifts like a brick in a building; one or another brick in some buildings may be missing or faulty.

These systems require years of effort from a person who wishes to help himself. Some of them even require him to devote his entire life to it.

Improvement of processes, as opposed to improvement of properties

This static approach turns correction into a lengthy and complicated process. I believe that it is based on wrong assumptions, for it is impossible to repair the faulty bricks in man's structure or to replace those which are missing. Man's life is a continuous process, and the improvement is needed in the quality of the process, not in his properties or disposition.

Many factors influence this process, and they must be combined to make it fluid and self-adjusting. The more clearly the fundamentals of the process are understood, the greater will be the achievements.

Faults are used in improvement

Just as in any complicated process deviations are used to help correct its progression, so in the correction of man faults and deviations should not be suppressed, overlooked, or overcome by force in any way, but used to direct his correction.

Correction of movements is the best means of self-improvement

It has been noted that any one of the four components of the waking state inescapably influences the others. The choice of movement as the main means of improving the self is based on the following reasoning:

1. The nervous system is occupied mainly with movement

Movement occupies the nervous system more than anything else because we cannot sense, feel, or think without a many-sided and elaborate series of actions initiated by the brain to maintain the body against the pull of gravity; at the same time we must know where we are and in what position. In order to know our position within the field of gravity with respect to other bodies or to change our position, we must make use of our senses, our feeling, and our power of thought.

The active involvement of the entire nervous system in the waking state is a part of every method of self-improvement, even in those that claim to be concerned with only one of the four components of the waking state.

2. It is easier to distinguish the quality of movement

We know more clearly and certainly about the organization of the body against the pull of gravity than we do about the other components. We know much more about movement than about anger, love, envy, or even thought. It is relatively easier to learn to recognize the quality of a movement than the quality of the other factors.

3. We have a richer experience of movement

We all have more experience of movement, and more capacity for it, than of feeling and thought. Many people do not differentiate between overexcitability and sensitivity, and consider highly developed sensitivity a weakness; they suppress any troubling feelings and avoid situations that might arouse such feelings. In a similar way thought is also restrained or broken off by many people. Freedom of thought is considered defiance of the accepted laws of behavior, not only in religion, but also in matters affecting ethnic affiliation, economics, morality, sex, art, politics, and even science.

4. The ability to move is important to self-value

A person's physical build and his ability to move are probably more important to his self-image than anything else. We must only watch a child who has found some imperfection in his mouth or something else in his appearance that seems to make him different from other children to convince ourselves that this discovery will affect his behavior considerably. If, for instance, his spine has not developed normally, he will have difficulty with movements requiring a keen sense of balance. He will stumble easily and will require a constant conscious effort to achieve what other children do quite naturally. He has developed differently from the others; he discovers that he must think and prepare himself in advance; he cannot rely on his own spontaneous reactions. Thus difficulties in moving undermine and distort his self-regard and force him into behavior that interferes with his development in the direction of his natural inclinations.

5. All muscular activity is movement

Every action originates in muscular activity. Seeing, talking, and even hearing require muscular action. (In hearing, the muscle regulates the tension of the eardrum in accordance with the loudness of the sound perceived.)

Not only are mechanical coordination and temporal and spatial accuracy important in every movement, its intensity is also important. Permanent relaxation of muscles causes action to be slow and feeble, and permanent excessive tension causes jerky and angular movements; both make states of mind apparent and are linked with the motive of the actions. Thus, in mental patients, nervous persons, and those with an unstable self-image, it is possible to discern disturbances in the muscular tonus in accordance with the deficiency. At the same time, other attributes of action, such as rhythm and adjustment in time and space, may be more satisfactory. It is possible to discern trouble in the regulation of intensity in movements and in the facial expression of a person on the street, even for an unskilled observer who does not know exactly what is wrong.

6. Movements reflect the state of the nervous system

The muscles contract as a result of an unending series of impulses from the nervous system; for this reason the muscular pattern of the upright position, facial expression, and voice reflect the condition of the nervous system. Obviously, neither position, expression, nor voice can be changed without a change in the nervous system that mobilizes the outward and visible changes.

Thus, when we refer to muscular movement, we mean, in fact, the impulses of the nervous system that activate the muscles, which cannot function without impulses to direct them. Though the heart muscle of the embryo begins to contract even before the nerves that will control it have developed, it does not work in the way familiar to us until its own nervous system can regulate its action. From this we may derive a conclusion that seems paradoxical at first sight: Improvement in action and movement will appear only after a prior change in the brain and the nervous system has occurred. That is, an improvement in body action reflects the change in the central control, which is the exclusive authority. The change in the center control is a change in the nervous system. As such, changes are invisible to the eye, their external expression is therefore considered as purely mental by some people, while others will consider them as purely physical.

7. Movement is the basis of awareness

Most of what goes on within us remains dulled and hidden from us until it reaches the muscles. We know what is happening within us as soon as the muscles of our face, heart, or breathing apparatus organize themselves into patterns, known to us as fear, anxiety, laughter, or any other feeling. Even though only a very short time is required to organize the muscular expression to the internal response or feeling, we all know that it is possible to check one's own laughter before it becomes noticeable to others. Similarly, we can prevent ourselves from giving visible expression to fear and other feelings.

We do not become aware of what is happening in our central nervous system until we become aware of changes that have taken place in our stance, stability, and attitude, for these changes are more easily felt than those that have occurred in the muscles themselves. We are able to prevent full muscular expression because the processes in that part of the brain that deals with functions peculiar to man alone are far slower than the processes in those parts of the brain dealing with what is common to both man and animals. It is the very slowness of these processes that makes it possible for us to judge and decide whether or not to act. The whole system ranges itself so that the muscles are ordered and ready either to carry out the action, or prevent it from being carried out.

As soon as we become aware of the means used to organize an expression, we may occasionally discern the stimulus that set it all off. In other words, we recognize the stimulus for an action, or the cause for a response, when we become sufficiently aware of the organization of the muscles of the body for the action concerned. Sometimes we may be aware that something is happening within us without being able to define exactly what it is. In this case a new pattern of organization is taking place and we do not yet know how to interpret it. When it has occurred several times it will become familiar; we will recognize its cause and sense the very first signs of the process. In some cases the experience will have to be repeated many times before it is recognized. Ultimately, we become aware of most of what is going on within us mainly through the muscles. A smaller part of this information reaches us through the envelope, that is, the skin that encompasses the whole body, the membranes that line the digestive tract, and the membranes that enclose and line the breathing organs and those of the inner surfaces of the mouth, nose, and the anus.

8. Breathing is movement

Our breathing reflects every emotional or physical effort and every disturbance. It is also sensitive to the vegetative processes. Disturbances of the thyroid gland, for instance, cause a special kind of breathing that serves to diagnose this disease. Any strong sudden stimulus causes a halt in breathing. Everybody knows from his own experience how closely linked breathing is with every change of feeling or anticipation of a strong emotion.

Throughout the history of mankind we find systems and rules designed to induce a calming effect by improved breathing. The human skeleton is so constructed that it is almost impossible to organize breathing properly without also satisfactorily placing the skeleton with respect to gravity. The reorganization of breathing alone succeeds only to the degree that we succeed indirectly in improving the organization of the skeletal muscles for better standing and better movement.

9. Hinges of habit

Finally, and most important of all, there is one more reason why we should choose the action-system as the point of attack for the improvement of man. All behavior, as we noted before, is a complex of mobilized muscles, sensing, feeling, and thought. Each of these components of action could, in theory, be used instead, but the part played by the muscles is so large in the alternatives that if it were omitted from the patterns in the motor cortex the rest of the components of the pattern would disintegrate.

The motor cortex of the brain, where patterns activating the muscles are established, lies only a few millimeters above the brain strata dealing with association processes. All the feeling and sensing that a man has experienced were at one time linked with the association processes.

The nervous system has a fundamental characteristic: We cannot carry out an action and its opposite at the same time. At any single moment the whole system achieves a kind of general integration that the body will express at that moment. Position, sensing, feeling, thought, as well as chemical and hormonal processes, combine to form a whole that cannot be separated out into its various parts. This whole may be highly complex and complicated, but is the integrated whole of the system at that given moment.

Within every such integration we become aware of only those

elements that involve the muscles and the envelope. We have already seen that the muscles play the main role in awareness. It is not possible for change to take place in the muscle system without a prior corresponding change in the motor cortex. If we can succeed in some way in bringing about a change in the motor cortex, and through this a change in the coordination of or in the patterns themselves, the basis of awareness in each elementary integration will disintegrate.

Owing to the close proximity to the motor cortex of the brain structures dealing with thought and feeling, and the tendency of processes in brain tissue to diffuse and spread to neighboring tissues, a drastic change in the motor cortex will have parallel effects on thinking and feeling.

A fundamental change in the motor basis within any single integration pattern will break up the cohesion of the whole and thereby leave thought and feeling without anchorage in the patterns of their established routines. In this condition it is much easier to effect changes in thinking and feeling, for the muscular part through which thinking and feeling reach our awareness has changed and no longer expresses the patterns previously familiar to us. Habit has lost its chief support, that of the muscles, and has become more amenable to change.

Abstraction is exclusively human

We have said that the whole life process can be broken down into four components: movement, sensing, feeling, and thought. The last element is different in most aspects from movement. We may perhaps accept the view that thought, in the form in which it is found in man, is specific to him. While some sparks of something similar to thought may, admittedly, be observed in the higher animals, there is no doubt that abstraction remains the exclusive province of man; the harmonic theory in music, space geometry, the theory of groups, or probability are unimaginable outside man's own mind. The human brain and nervous system also have a structural peculiarity in one part that is essentially different from the structures in other parts of the brain that are on the whole similar to those possessed by other living creatures. There is no space here for a detailed analysis of the anatomical and physiological differences, and a general description of its structure will have to suffice.

The strictly individual part of the brain

The brain requires a certain chemical environment and a certain temperature for subsistence. And every living body contains a group of structures that direct and regulate the chemistry and heat of the whole in such a way that it may survive. This group of structures is the Rhinic system; it supplies the individual internal requirements of every living organism. If these structures are faulty, the whole organism will be crippled or not viable at all. These structures are symmetrical and are inherited in every detail of arrangement and functioning.

Internal periodic drives

A second group of structures in the brain deal with everything that concerns the outward expression of vital internal needs. The need to sustain the body and the Rhinic system creates internal drives that express themselves toward the environment. This is done by the Lymbic system, a group of structures that deal with everything concerning the individual's movements in the field of gravity and the satisfaction of all internal drives, such as hunger and thirst and the elimination of waste products. In short, it deals with all internal needs that intensify when not satisfied, but that are reduced or abated when satisfied, until the need increases and the cycle starts again.

All the marvels that we usually call instinct, such as the building of nests by birds, the spider's web, and the ability of the bee and the pigeon to find their way home over great distances, originate in these structures.

The dawn of the ability to learn

In activities of this kind the specific properties of the human nervous system are already noticeable. The structure, organization, and actions are mainly inherited, by contrast with the Rhinic system described above, which is entirely inherited and remains unchanged from individual to individual, except in cases of basic evolutionary changes.

Instincts are not as stationary and definite as we often think; they vary, and there are small instinctual differences between individuals. In some cases the instinct is weak, and a certain amount of individual experience is needed for action to proceed, as where, for instance, a newborn child fails to suck until its lips are stimulated with the nipple. In some cases, instinct permits a fair degree of adjustment to circumstances and the first hint of ability to change with a changing environment is found—in short, the birth or dawn of the ability to learn. Thus, for instance, birds accustom themselves to building nests of new materials when they are moved to strange surroundings. But the adjustment is difficult, and not all individuals succeed equally well; some do not manage to adjust at all. The adjustment of instincts to the demands of new surroundings may go so far as to approach what we are accustomed to call understanding and learning.

Fine differentiation is a human prerogative

A third group of structures of the brain is concerned with activities that distinguish man from animals. This is the Supralymbic system, which is much more highly developed in man than in any of the higher animals. It is this system that assures the delicate differentiation of the muscles of the hand, thereby multiplying the possible number of patterns, rhythms, and shades of any operation. This system turns the human hand into an instrument capable of playing music, drawing, writing, or doing many other activities. The Supralymbic system imparts an equal sensitivity to the muscles of the mouth, throat, and breathing apparatus. Similarly, here the power of differentiation multiplies the number of different sound patterns that it is possible to produce, resulting in the creation of hundreds of languages and a great variety of ways of singing and whistling.

Individual experience versus heredity

The structure and tissues of this nerve system are inherited, but their function depends largely on individual experience. No two handwritings are alike. An individual's handwriting will depend on the language he first learned to write, the kind of writing he was taught, the pen or other instrument he used, the position taken up while writing, and so on; that is, it will depend on everything that affected the formation of patterns or codes in the motor cortex of the brain while learning.

The proper pronunciation of an individual's mother tongue largely determines the development of the muscles of his tongue, mouth, voice, and his palate. A man's first language will affect the relative strength of the muscles of his mouth and the structure of the cavity to such an extent that in any subsequent language spoken it will be possible to recognize what language the person spoke before, owing to the difficulty of adjusting the organs of speech to the new inflections. Here the individual's personal experience actually becomes a factor that determines the structural development no less than the hereditary factors themselves. This is a unique peculiarity.

The concept of opposites derives from structure

The activity in the third system is asymmetrical—the right side differs from the left side—as opposed to the symmetry that is the rule in the other two systems. This asymmetry is behind the differentiation of right and left. When the right hand is dominant, the speech center forms on the left side of the brain and inversely. It is assumed that this primary opposition between right and left is the basis of our concept of opposites in general. As the right hand is usually the more functional one, in many languages the word "right" also carries such meanings as correct, law, a claim to something, and authority; for example, note the English "right," the Russian "pravo," the German "recht," and the French "droit."

Primitive modes of thought tend to oppose good to bad, black to white, cold to hot, light to dark, and to see in them opposition or conflict. More developed thinking can hardly attribute opposition to them in any real sense. Dark and cold, for instance, are by no means the opposites of light and heat: where there is no light it is dark; and the relationship between heat and cold is even more complicated.

Reversible and irreversible phenomena

The link with the centers of emotion is considerably weaker in this third system compared with the stronger links of the two previous ones. Strong emotions, such as anger or jealousy, interfere with the operation of this new, delicate system and confuse thought. But thought that is not connected to feeling at all is not connected to reality. Cerebration itself is uncommitted or neutral, and can deal equally well with contradictory statements. In order to select a thought there must at least be the feeling that the thought is "right," that is, it corresponds to reality. The rightness in this case is, of course, a subjective reality. When "right" objectively corresponds to reality, the thought will be of general human value.

Cerebration alone cannot decide between the two statements: "It is possible to get to the moon" and "It is not possible to get to the moon," for both statements are acceptable in themselves. The experience of reality alone endows a thought with the property of "right." For many generations reality disproved the former statement, and to "live on the moon" was said to indicate that the speaker's mind is divorced from reality.

Where pure cerebration is concerned, most processes could as easily be reversible as nonreversible. In reality the great majority of processes are irreversible: A match that has been struck and burned cannot revert back to a match; a tree cannot revert back to a sapling.

Processes connected with time are irreversible because time itself is irreversible. Indeed, few processes of any kind are reversible, that is, can retrace their steps so that the condition that existed before the process took place is restored. Cerebration not connected with reality does not constitute thought, any more than random muscular contractions constitute action or movement.

The delay between thought and action is the basis for awareness

The nerve paths in the third brain system are longer and more elaborate than in the two older systems. Most of the operations of the third system are carried out through the agency of the other two, although there are paths for the third system to exercise direct control over the executing mechanisms. The indirect process causes delay in the action itself, so that "Think first, act later" is not just a saying.

There is a delay between what is engendered in the Supralymbic system and its execution by the body. This delay between a thought process and its translation into action is long enough to make it possible to inhibit it. This possibility of creating the image of an action and then delaying its execution—postponing it or preventing it altogether—is the basis of imagination and intellectual judgment.

Most of the actions of this system are carried out by the older systems, and their speed is limited to that of the older ones. Thus, for instance, it is not possible to apprehend the meaning of printed matter faster than the eye can travel across the page to read it. Thought cannot be expressed more quickly than it can be pronounced in words. It follows that faster reading and faster expression are one of the means to faster thinking.

The possibility of a pause between the creation of the thought pattern for any particular action and the execution of that action is the physical basis for awareness. This pause makes it possible to examine what is happening within us at the moment when the intention to act is formed as well as when it is carried out. The possibility of delaying action—prolonging the period between the intention and its execution—enables man to learn to know himself. And there is much to know, for the systems that carry out our internal drives act automatically, as they do in the rest of the higher animals.

Doing does not mean knowing

The execution of an action by no means proves that we know, even superficially, what we are doing or how we are doing it. If we attempt to carry out an action with awareness—that is, to follow it in detail— we soon discover that even the simplest and most common of actions, such as getting up from a chair, is a mystery, and that we have no idea at all of how it is done: Do we contract the muscles of the stomach or of the back, do we tense the legs first, or tilt the body forward first; what do the eyes do, or the head? It is easy to demonstrate that man does not know what he is doing, right down to being unable to rise from a chair. He therefore has no choice but to return to his accustomed method, which is to give himself the order to get up and to leave it to the specialized organizations within himself to carry out the action as it pleases them, which means as he usually does.

We may thus learn that self-knowledge does not come without considerable effort, and can even interfere with the carrying out of actions. Thought and the intellect that knows are the enemies of automatic, habitual action. This fact is illustrated in the old story of the centipede who forgot how to walk after he had been asked in what order he moved all his multitude of legs.

Awareness fits action to intention

It is often enough for a man who is doing something to simply ask himself what he is doing in order for him to become confused and unable to continue. In such a case he has suddenly realized that the performance of the action does not really correspond to what he thought he was doing. Without awakened awareness we perform what the older brain systems do in their own way, even though the intention to act came from the higher third system. Moreover, the action often enough proves to be the exact opposite of the original intention. This happens when the intention to act comes from the higher system, whose link with the emotions is weak, and triggers into action the lower systems, which have much stronger links with the emotions because of the greater speed and also shortens delay between intention and performance.

In such cases the faster automatic and quicker action of the lower brain systems causes that part of the action that is related to more intense feeling to be carried out almost immediately, while the part that relates to thought (coming from the higher system) will come in slowly, when the action is almost completed or even over. Most slips of the tongue arise in this fashion.

Awareness is not essential to life

The two older systems, the Rhinic and the Lymbic, are harmoniously adjusted to each other in most people. These two systems can satisfy essential human needs and perform all man's actions, including those we attribute to intelligence. Even social life is not impossible without the Supralymbic system, as highly developed as it is in the human animal. Bees, ants, monkeys, and herd animals live in social systems without awareness. Some of these social systems are fairly elaborate and involve most of the basic functions of human society: the care of the younger generation, rule by a king, wars with neighbors, defense of home territory, the exploitation of slaves, and other joint actions.

Awareness as a new stage in evolution

The upper system, which is more highly developed in man than in any other animal, makes awareness possible, that is, recognition of organic needs and the selection of means for their satisfaction. Thanks to the nature of this system, awareness gives us the capacity for judgment, differentiation, generalization, the capacity for abstract thought, imagination, and much more. Awareness of our organic drives is the basis of man's self-knowledge. Awareness of the relationship between these impulses and their origin in the formation of human culture offers man the potential means to direct his life, which few people have yet realized.

I believe that we are living in a historically brief transition period that heralds the emergence of the truly human man.

The Direction
of Progress

Every man has two worlds: a personal world of his own and the external world common to us all. In my personal world, the universe and all living things exist only as long as I live; my world is born with me and dies and disappears together with me. In the great world we all share I am no more than a drop of water in the sea or a grain of sand in the desert. My life and death hardly affect the great world at all.

The aim of a man in life is his private affair, up to a point. One man dreams of happiness, another of wealth, a third of power, a fourth of knowledge or justice, and still others of equality. But we do not even begin to know the purpose of mankind as such. The only idea that has a reasonable basis and that is accepted by all the sciences is that there is a direction in the development of living creatures, and that man stands at the top of the ladder of this development. This direction of evolution may also be interpreted as its purpose. We saw this purpose in detailing the structures of our own nervous system in the previous chapter. There, the direction of development was toward increasing the capacity of awareness to direct older processes and actions developed during earlier evolutionary periods, to increase their variety, to inhibit them, or to speed them up. We ourselves realize this trend inadvertently when we

observe that some artist or scientist may be very able but that there is
something missing that would make him fully "human."

Consciousness and awareness

All the more highly developed animals have a considerable amount
of consciousness. They know the surroundings in which they live and
their place within the family group, herd, or flock. They can cooperate
for the defense of the family or herd and even help a member of their
tribe, which means that they perhaps recognize what is good for their
neighbor. Man is endowed with not only a more highly developed
consciousness but with a specific capacity for abstraction that enables
him to discriminate and to know what is happening within him when
he uses this power. Thus he may know whether he does or does not know
something. He can tell whether he does or does not understand something he knows. He is capable of a still higher form of abstraction that
enables him to estimate his power of abstraction and the extent to which
he uses it. He can tell whether he is using his full powers of awareness
in order to know, and whether he realizes that he does not know something.

There is an essential difference between consciousness and awareness,
although the borders are not clear in our use of language. I can walk up
the stairs of my house, fully conscious of what I am doing, and yet not
know how many steps I have climbed. In order to know how many there
are I must climb them a second time, pay attention, listen to myself,
and count them. Awareness is consciousness together with a realization
of what is happening within it or of what is going on within ourselves
while we are conscious.

Many people find it easy to be aware of control of their voluntary
muscles, thought, and abstraction processes. It is much more difficult, on the other hand, to be aware and in control of the involuntary muscles, senses, emotions, and creative abilities. Despite this
difficulty, it is by no means impossible, even though this seems unlikely to many.

We act as a whole entity even when this wholeness is not quite perfect. From this springs the possibility of also developing awareness control in the more difficult parts. The changes that occur in the parts where control is easy also affect the rest of the system, including those parts over which we have no direct power. Indirect influence is also a kind of control. Our work is a method of training that converts this initial indirect influence into clear knowledge.

It should perhaps be made explicit at this point that we are speaking of the training of will power and self-control, but not for the purpose of gaining power over ourselves or over other people. Correction of the self, improvement, training of awareness, and other concepts have been used here to describe various aspects of the idea of development. Development stresses the harmonious coordination between structure, function, and achievement. And a basic condition for harmonious coordination is complete freedom from either self-compulsion or compulsion from others.

Normal development in general is harmonious. In development the parts grow, improve, and strengthen in such a way that the whole can continue toward its general destination. And just as new functions appear in the course of a child's harmonious development and growth, so do new powers appear in any harmonious development.

Harmonious development is not a simple matter. Let us take, for instance, abstract thought, which at first sight seems to be wholly an advantage; concerning harmonious development, however, it also has many disadvantages. Abstraction is the basis of verbalization. Words symbolize the meanings they describe and could not be created without the abstraction of the quality or character of the thing represented. It is difficult to imagine any human culture whatsoever without words. Abstract thought and verbalization occupy the most important place in science and in all social achievement. But at the same time abstraction and verbalization become a tyrant who deprives the individual of concrete reality; this, in turn, causes severe disturbances in the harmony of most human activities. Frequently the degree of disturbance borders on mental and physical illness and causes premature senility. As verbal abstraction becomes more successful and more efficient, man's thinking and imagination become further estranged from his feelings, senses, and even movements.

We have seen that the structures used for thinking are loosely linked with those housing feeling. Clear thought is born only in the absence of strong feelings that distort objectivity. Thus a necessary condition for the development of effective thinking is continuous withdrawal from feelings and proprioceptive sensations.

Nevertheless, harmonious development remains more important to the individual than discordant development even if effective thinking is the disturbing factor. Thinking that is cut off from the rest of the man gradually becomes arid. Thought that proceeds mainly in words does not draw substance from the processes of the older evolutionary structures that are closely tied to feeling. Creative, spontaneous thought must maintain a link with the early brain structures. Abstract thought that is not nourished from time to time from deeper sources within us becomes a fabric of words alone, empty of all genuine human content. Many books of art and science, literature and poetry have nothing to offer except a succession of words linked together by logical argument; they have no personal content. This also applies to many individuals in their daily relationships with others. Thinking that does not develop harmoniously with the rest of man becomes an obstacle to his proper development.

It may seem to be a somewhat trivial conclusion that harmonious development is a desirable thing. As long as we consider only the abstractions and logical content of this phrase it will remain divorced from the "whole man" like any other piece of logical verbalization, without practical significance. The trivial phrase will, however, become an unlimited source of forms, figures, and relationships that make new combinations and discoveries possible only when we stimulate our emotions and senses and direct impressions—that is, when we think in images, in our varied mental combinations. It is these that must be clothed in words in order to establish human contact with our fellows.

Harmonious development is found in every creature whose species has a long history. This kind of development is accompanied by many difficulties in the case of man because of the relative newness of awareness in the evolutionary ladder. The harmonious development of animals, anthropoids, and of the earliest man require senses, feelings, movement, and only a minimum of thought, which is memory and a little consciousness—all that is necessary to make the waking condition different from sleep.

Animals without awareness wander here and there without any further significance. When awareness appeared on the evolutionary ladder in man, a simple movement in one direction became a turn to the left, in the other direction a turn to the right.

It is difficult for us to appreciate the significance of this fact; it seems a simple matter to us, just as the power of seeing seems simple to our eyes. But a little thought will show us that, in fact, the power to differentiate between right and left is no less complicated than sight. When man differentiates between right and left he divides space with respect to himself, taking himself as the center from which this space extends. This sense of a division in space, which is not yet altogether clear in our awareness, is often expressed as "on the right hand" and "on the left hand." This provides a further abstraction in the concepts of "right" and "left" that can thus now be expressed in words. In time the symbols become increasingly abstract and it becomes possible to construct such sentences as this one. To achieve a tiny step forward in awareness, such as the understanding of right and left, man must at one time have paid attention as he moved, alternately to what went on inside him and in the world outside. This shifting of the attention inward and outward creates abstractions and words that describe the shift in the position of his personal world relative to the outer world. Clearly the development of this awareness is bound up with considerable birth pangs, and the first glimmerings of awareness must have bewildered our ancestors many times.

Owing to its newness in an evolutionary sense, the degree of awareness differs greatly between different individuals, far more than the relative distribution of other faculties. Further, there are also great periodic variations in the individual's awareness and its value relative to other aspects of his personality. There may be a low point at which awareness may disappear momentarily or for a period. More rarely there may be a high point at which there is a harmonious unity, with all man's capacities fused into a single whole.

In the esoteric schools of thought a Tibetan parable is told. According to the story, a man without awareness is like a carriage whose passengers are the desires, with the muscles for horses, while the carriage itself is the skeleton. Awareness is the sleeping coachman. As long as the coachman remains asleep the carriage will be dragged aimlessly here and there. Each passenger seeks a different destination and the horses pull different ways. But when the coachman is wide awake and holds the reins the horses will pull the carriage and bring every passenger to his proper destination.

In those moments when awareness succeeds in being at one with feeling, senses, movement, and thought, the carriage will speed along on the right road. Then man can make discoveries, invent, create, innovate, and "know." He grasps that his small world and the great world around are but one and that in this unity he is no longer alone.

PART TWO

Doing to Understand: Twelve Practical Lessons

These twelve lessons have been selected from among more than a thousand given over the years at the Feldenkrais Institute. The lessons do not represent a sequence, but were chosen rather to illustrate points from the author's system and the technique used to convey it. They nevertheless represent exercises involving the whole body and its essential activities.

Students attempting these lessons should do one every evening immediately before going to sleep. Within a few weeks they will find a considerable improvement in all functions essential to life.

General Observations

Improvement of ability

The lessons are designed to improve ability, that is, to expand the boundaries of the possible: to turn the impossible into the possible, the difficult into the easy, and the easy into the pleasant. For only those activities that are easy and pleasant will become part of a man's habitual life and will serve him at all times. Actions that are hard to carry out, for which man must force himself to overcome his inner opposition, will never become part of his normal daily life; as he gets older he will lose his ability to carry them out at all.

It is rare, for instance, for a man over fifty to jump over a fence, even if it is quite low. He will look for the way around the fence, while a youth will jump over it without any difficulty.

This does not mean that we should avoid everything that seems difficult and never use our will power to overcome obstacles, but that we should differentiate clearly between improvement of ability and sheer effort for its own sake. We shall do better to direct our will power to improving our ability so that in the end our actions will be carried out easily and with understanding.

Ability and will power

To the extent that ability increases, the need for conscious efforts of the will decreases. The effort required to increase ability provides sufficient and efficient exercise for our will power. If you consider the matter carefully you will discover that most people of strong will power (which they have trained for its own sake) are also people with relatively poor ability. People who know how to operate effectively do so without great preparation and without much fuss. Men of great will power tend to apply too much force instead of using moderate forces more effectively.

If you rely mainly on your will power, you will develop your ability to strain and become accustomed to applying an enormous amount of force to actions that can be carried out with much less energy, if it is properly directed and graduated.

Both these ways of operating usually achieve their objective, but the former may also cause considerable damage. Force that is not converted into movement does not simply disappear, but is dissipated into damage done to joints, muscles, and other sections of the body used to create the effort. Energy not converted into movement turns into heat within the system and causes changes that will require repair before the system can operate efficiently again.

Whatever we can do well does not seem difficult to us. We may even venture to say that movements we find difficult are not carried out correctly.

To understand movement we must feel, not strain

To learn we need time, attention, and discrimination; to discriminate we must sense. This means that in order to learn we must sharpen our powers of sensing, and if we try to do most things by sheer force we shall achieve precisely the opposite of what we need.

When learning to act we should be free to pay attention to what is going on inside us, for in this condition our mind will be clear and breathing easy to control; there is no tension engendered by stress. When learning is carried out under conditions of maximum effort, and even this does not seem enough, there is no longer any way of speeding up action or making it stronger or better, because the individual has already reached the limit of his capacity. At this point breathing is arrested; there is superfluous effort, little ability to observe, and no prospect of improvement.

In the course of the lessons the reader will find that the exercises suggested are in themselves simple, involving only easy movements. But they are intended to be carried out in such a way that those who do them will discover changes in themselves even after the first lesson.

Sharpened discrimination

"A fool cannot feel," said the Hebrew sages. If a man does not feel he cannot sense differences, and of course he will not be able to distinguish between one action and another. Without this ability to differentiate there can be no learning, and certainly no increase in the ability to learn. It is not a simple matter, for the human senses are linked to the stimuli that produce them so that discrimination is finest when the stimulus is smallest.

If I raise an iron bar I shall not feel the difference if a fly either lights on it or leaves it. If, on the other hand, I am holding a feather, I shall feel a distinct difference if the fly were to settle on it. The same applies to all the senses: hearing, sight, smell, taste, heat, and cold.

The exercises here are intended to reduce effort in movement, for in order to recognize small changes in effort, the effort itself must first be reduced. More delicate and improved control of movement is possible only through the increase of sensitivity, through a greater ability to sense differences.

The force of habit

It is extremely difficult to correct a faulty habit of posture or movement even if it has been clearly recognized. For both the fault and the
way in which it appears in action must be corrected. We need a great
deal of persistence and enough knowledge to enable us to move according to what we know rather than according to habit.

If a person usually stands with his stomach and pelvis pushed too far
forward, with his head tilted back as a result, there will be far too great
a curve in his back for good posture. If he then brings his head forward
and pushes his pelvis back he will have the feeling that his head is
actually tilted to the front and his pelvis too far back; and the position
will seem to him abnormal. As a result he will quickly return to his
habitual stance.

It is therefore impossible to change habit by relying on sensation
alone. Some conscious mental effort must be made until the adjusted
position ceases to feel abnormal and becomes the new habit. It is much
more difficult to change a habit than one might think, as all who have
ever tried know.

Thinking while acting

In my lessons the student learns to listen to the instructions while he
is actually carrying out an exercise and to make the necessary adjustments without stopping the movement itself. *In this way he learns to act
while he thinks and to think while he acts.* This is a step up in the ladder
of ability from the man who stops thinking while he does something and
stops acting when he wants to think. (An experienced driver can easily
carry out instructions while he is driving, while a beginner has difficulty
doing this.)

In order to obtain maximum benefit from these exercises, the reader
must therefore try to project the instructions for the next exercise

without stopping the previous one; he must continue the movement he is performing while preparing his thoughts for the next one.

Freeing an action of wasted energy

An efficient machine is one in which all the parts fit together accurately; all are properly oiled, with no grit or dirt between adjacent surfaces; where all the fuel used is turned into kinetic energy up to the thermodynamic limit; and where there is no noise or vibration, that is, no energy is wasted on useless movement that cuts down the effective operating power of the machine.

The exercises we are about to begin are intended to achieve just this, to gradually eliminate from one's mode of action all superfluous movements, everything that hampers, interferes with, or opposes movement.

In the systems of teaching generally accepted today emphasis is placed on achieving a certain aim at any price, without regard for the amount of disorganized and diffused effort that has gone into it. So long as the organs of thought, feeling, and control are not organized for action that is coordinated, continuous, smooth, and efficient—and therefore also pleasant—we are involving parts of the body indiscriminately, even if they are in no way required for this action or even interfere with it. One result is that we quite often perform an action and its opposite at the same time. Only mental effort can then make the part that is directed toward the goal overcome the other parts of the body operating to frustrate it. In this way, unfortunately, *will power may tend to cover up an inability* to carry out the action properly. The right way is to learn to eliminate the efforts opposing the goal and to employ will power only when a superhuman effort is required.

We shall come back to this point when the reader has proved it to himself through his own experience; he will then be able to progress further along the desired road.

Breathing rhythm during the exercises

At the end of a lesson that has been properly carried out, you should feel fresh and relaxed as after a good sleep or a holiday. If this does not happen, the movements were probably made too quickly and without attention to breathing.

The speed of the exercise should always be adjusted to the breathing rhythm. As the body gains in organization, breathing will automatically adjust itself to the various movements.

Speed of movements

The first time you attempt a lesson it should be carried out as slowly as the instructions indicate. After you have finished all the lessons and go through them a second time, you should go faster in those parts that are smooth and easy. Subsequently you should vary the speed from as fast as possible to as slow as possible.

Some
Practical
Hints

When to exercise

The best time to exercise is just before going to bed at night, but at least an hour after dinner. Go to bed as soon as you have finished. One of the most important reasons for this is that after a day of work and worry the exercises will relieve both mental and muscular tension and sleep will be more restful and refreshing.

When you wake up, stretch for a minute or more in bed, and try to recall the general feeling of the lesson you did the night before. It is worthwhile to repeat two or three of the movements that you can remember. Think over the lesson from time to time during the day while you are doing other things, and see whether you can identify any changes it has caused.

Set yourself fixed times for this during the day, even if it is only for a few seconds at a time. Every time that you recall the past lesson it will become more firmly established in your mind.

When the exercises have become an established daily habit, do them at whatever time is most convenient.

Duration of the exercises

The time the lesson takes to do will depend on individual speed. In the early lessons the number of times each movement is repeated will more or less decide the amount of time. Start by repeating each movement 10 times; as you progress increase the number to 25, in accordance with the instructions given in the lesson itself. In time it is possible and desirable to repeat a single movement hundreds of times, both as slowly as possible and as fast as possible. But remember that fast does not mean hurried.

From this we see that the early lessons will take about 45 minutes each to carry out, the later ones may take only 20 minutes or so; after that, when exercising becomes a daily routine, a lesson may take from a moment's time for thinking up to whatever time the individual chooses to spend on it.

Where to exercise

Choose an area of floor covered with a carpet or mat that is large enough to allow you to stretch out your arms and legs sideways without being hemmed in by furniture or other objects. If you have trouble at first getting used to lying on the floor, use a thick blanket or work on a bed if necessary.

What to wear

The less you wear the better. In any case make sure that whatever you wear is comfortable and does not interfere with your movements or breathing, that it is not too tight, and has no buttons or slide fasteners at the back.

THE BODY MIND CONNECTION LTD
914 KING STREET
ALEXANDRIA, VA   22314
703-519-8644
THANK YOU!

DATE: 12/10/97   TIME: 16:54:31
MERH: 064300080107 STR#: 3010 TERM: 0001

S-A-L-E-S D-R-A-F-T

REF: 3213
BATCH=   555
CD TYPE: MAST
TR TYPE= PR

AMOUNT= $12.54

TOTAL= $12.54

ACCT: 5434024472671195   EXP: 0399
AP: 010815
NAME: MRS G GROSVENOR

X_____

TOP COPY-MERCHANT BOTTOM COPY-CUSTOMER

How to do the lessons

If you are working alone and must read the instructions yourself, it is best to do a small part at a time. Read a short paragraph of the instructions, enough to tell you what you should do, and begin. When you have repeated the movement 25 times, as instructed, read the next paragraph and carry it out. In this way go through the lesson paragraph by paragraph. The lesson will take longer this way, so it is best to divide it up into sections and do it in installments. When you have learned all the movements in a lesson and no longer need the instructions, put the sections together and do the whole lesson in one.

What is
Good Posture?

Standing properly is not straight

"Sit straight!" "Stand straight!" This is often said by mothers, teachers, and others who give this directive in good faith and the fullest confidence in what they are saying. If you were to ask them just how one does sit or stand straight, they would answer, "What do you mean? Don't you know what straight means? Straight is straight!"

Some people do indeed stand and walk straight, with their backs erect and their heads held high. And of course there is an element of "standing straight" in their posture.

If you watch a child or an adult who has been told to sit or stand straight, it is evident that he agrees that there is something wrong with the way he is managing his body, and he will quickly try to straighten his back or raise his head. He will do this thinking that he has thereby achieved the proper posture; but he cannot maintain this "correct" position without a continuous effort. As soon as his attention shifts to some activity that is either necessary, urgent, or interesting, he will slump back to his original posture.

It is almost certain that he will not try to "hold himself straight" again unless he is reminded to do so, or unless he himself feels that he has neglected this instruction.

By straight we mean vertical

When we speak of standing straight in this sense we almost always mean vertical. But if we look at the ideal skeleton constructed by the famous anatomist Albinus, we shall find only two small sections that are ranged more or less vertically: the top vertebrae of the neck and the vertebrae between the chest and the hips. No other bone in the entire skeleton is placed in a precisely vertical direction (although the bones of the arms are sometimes held more or less vertically). Thus when we say straight we obviously mean something different, for we have no precise idea of the meaning of the word in this connection.

Straight is an aesthetic concept

The word "straight" is misleading. It does not express what is needed, nor even what we expect to achieve or see after improvement has taken place. "Straight" is used in a purely aesthetic sense in connection with posture, and as such is neither useful nor precise, thus it will not serve as a criterion for the correction of faults.

Nor will the geometrical sense of straight serve any better, because it is static. Whatever part of the body is to be straight could comply with the geometrical sense of the word by being held motionless in the same position, without any change.

To appreciate fully how little the accepted meaning of straight coincides with what is right in posture we have only to consider the case of a man who has broken his back and is unable to straighten it. How shall he stand or sit? Can a disabled person really not use his body properly, efficiently, and gracefully? There are many cripples whose ability in this respect surpasses that of healthy people. There are persons who have suffered severe damage to their bone structure and yet the power, accuracy, and grace of their movements are outstanding. But the concept of straight simply cannot be applied to them at all.

Skeleton, muscles, and gravity

It follows that any posture is acceptable in itself as long as it does not conflict with the law of nature, which is that the skeletal structure should counteract the pull of gravity, leaving the muscles free for movement. The nervous system and the frame develop together under the influence of gravity in such a way that the skeleton will hold up the body without expending energy despite the pull of gravity. If, on the other hand, the muscles have to carry out the job of the skeleton, not only do they use energy needlessly, but they are then prevented from carrying out their main function of changing the position of the body, that is, of movement.

In poor posture the muscles are doing a part of the job of the bones. In order to correct posture it is important to discover what has distorted the reaction of the nervous system to gravity, to which every part of the whole system has had to adjust as long as man has existed.

In order to arrive at any practical understanding of this problem we will have to examine and clarify the concepts used above. Let us first see what is the correct response of the system to gravity.

Relaxation: a concept that is often misunderstood

Let us look at the lower half of the jaw. Most people keep their mouths closed when they are not speaking, eating, or doing something else with it. What keeps the lower half of the jaw drawn up against the upper half? If the relaxation that has now become so fashionable were the correct condition, then the lower jaw would hang down freely and the mouth remain wide open. But this ultimate state of relaxation is found only among individuals born idiots, or in cases of paralyzing shocks.

It is important to understand how an essential part of the body such as the jaw can be in this permanent state of being held up, supported by muscles that work ceaselessly while we are awake; yet we do not sense that we are doing anything to hold up our jaw. In order to let our jaw drop freely we actually have to learn to inhibit the muscles involved. If you try to relax the lower jaw until its own weight opens the mouth fully you will find that it is not easy. When you have succeeded you will observe that there are also changes in the expression of the face and in the eyes. It is likely that you will discover at the end of this experiment that your jaw is normally shut too tightly.

Perhaps you will also discover the origin of this excessive tension. Watch for the return of the tension after the jaw has been relaxed, and you will at least discover how infinitely little man knows about his own powers and about himself in general.

The results of this small experiment can be important for a sensible person, more important even than attending to his business, because his ability to make a livelihood may improve when he discovers what is reducing the efficiency of most of his activities.

No awareness of action in antigravity muscles

The lower jaw is not the only part of the body that does not drop down as far as it can. The head itself does not drop forward. Its center of gravity is well in front of the point at which it is supported by the spine (it lies approximately between the ears), for the face and front part of the skull are heavier than the back of the head. Despite this structure the head does not fall forward, so obviously there must be some organization in the system that keeps it up.

If we relax the muscles at the back of the neck completely, then the head will drop to the lowest possible position, with the chin resting on the breastbone. Yet there is no consciousness of effort while these muscles at the back of the neck are contracted to hold up the head.

If you finger the calf muscles (at the back of the leg, at about the middle) while standing, you will find them strongly contracted. If they were entirely relaxed the body would fall forward. In good posture the bones of the lower leg are at a small angle forward from the vertical, and the contraction of the muscles of the calves prevents the body from falling forward on its face.

We stand without knowing how

We are thus not aware of any effort or activity in the muscles that work against gravity. We become aware of the antigravity muscles only when we either interrupt or reinforce them, that is , when the voluntary change is made in clear awareness. The permanent contraction that is normally present before any intentional act is done is not registered by our senses. The electrical impulses, which derive from different sources within the nervous system, are involved. One group of these produces deliberate action; the other group causes contraction in the antigravity muscles until the work done by them exactly balances the pull of gravity.

The upright posture is maintained by an old part of the nervous system

A study of the limbs and parts of the body, such as the shoulders, eyes, eyelids, and so on, shows that their muscles are constantly working, work that is not sensed and that is not due to any conscious effort. How many people are aware, for instance, that their eyelids are raised, and can feel their weight? This weight is felt only in the moments between wakefulness and sleep, when it suddenly becomes difficult to keep one's eyes open: that is, when a sudden effort is needed to do so. As long as we are upright, our eyelids will not fall despite their weight. The upright position and all that it involves is organized by a special section of the nervous system, which performs a great deal of complicated work of which no more than a hint penetrates into our conscious mind. This section is one of the oldest in the evolution of the human species; it is certainly older than the voluntary system, and it is also physically placed below it.

The link between instinct and intention

Good posture, then, should be the privilege of every person born without gross defects. Further, as the organization of this posture is carried out by a system that works automatically, independently of the individual's volition, all humans should stand upright in the same way, just as one cat stands like every other cat, and every sparrow flies in exactly the same way.

But reality is usually both simpler and more complex than it appears at first sight. We like to think that instinct is something totally different from knowledge and understanding. We believe that the bee and the spider and the other engineers of the animal kingdom perform by instinct and automatically, without any need to learn, the things that we do with the aid of our brain, consciousness, and will, and only after much elaborate study. This is only partly correct. Even instinct does not operate altogether automatically, and the things that we do deliberately are not totally divorced from instinct.

Man's capacity to learn replaces the instincts of the animals

Man's instincts have become feeble by comparison with those of animals. Not every infant begins to breathe the moment it is born, and sometimes vigorous action must be taken before a baby will draw its first breath. The same applies to sucking. Many infants have to be encouraged and stimulated before the first drive is aroused that will make them feel the urge and ability to satisfy a vital need. Man has no clear and unmistakable instincts to guide him either in walking or in other movements, and not even in sexual activity. His capacity for learning, on the other hand, is incomparably greater than that of any other living creature. The stronger instincts of the animals do not permit them to cease or resist instinctive action, and obviously change in an instinctive action is neither easy to achieve nor permanent.

Our ability to learn, therefore, which involves the developing of new responses to familiar stimuli as the result of experience, is man's special characteristic. It serves us in place of powerful instincts, where even the slightest changes come about only with great difficulty.

Man learns mainly from experience, animals mainly from the experience of their species

The function of speech will serve as a good example to help us understand our other functions. Every child born without some gross defect has the skeletal, muscular, and nervous equipment to allow him to learn to speak through hearing and imitating sounds. The animals with their stronger instincts, on the other hand, have little need to learn. Their executing mechanisms are linked almost from birth with the ordering mechanisms of the nervous system. The connections in the nervous sytem are predetermined and a minimum of experience is required to impress the function permanently.

The nightingale thus sings the same song in Japan and in Mexico. (This may not be absolutely, scientifically accurate, but it is close enough for our purpose.) Bees construct their hives according to the same pattern wherever they happen to live; and every animal in whose veins there is dog's blood will bark, even if it also has a share of wolf or jackal blood.

But in man there is no speech pattern that is fixed from birth; speech develops and grows anatomically, and at the same time functionally. A child will speak Chinese if he grows up in China; or he learns whatever language is appropriate to his surroundings. Wherever he happens to be, he will have to form through his personal experience the connections between the cells of his nervous system that activate the muscles he needs for speech.

At first these cells are provided only with the power to freely establish whatever combination of patterns experience will provide. These patterns, created by the individual's experience and not by the collective experience of the human race, are therefore permanent only as long as the experience is stable. It is even possible to forget one's mother tongue. And it is not very difficult to learn another language.

Individual experience

But it is the early attempts at speech that have the greatest influence on the development of the mouth and on the relative strength of the vocal cords. Every subsequent attempt at learning a new language will be hampered by the early influences and it will be more difficult to become accustomed to the new forms. Learning a new language is also made more difficult by the existing speech forms that impede new combinations of movements of the muscles of the mouth and throat, for they have already acquired a tendency to continue the former patterns automatically.

Man's greater power of adjustment

These observations will help us to understand why posture in standing and walking can be so different in different people, even though it is controlled by a part of the brain whose functions are closer to instinctual than voluntary action.

Upright posture, like speech, has no ready-made connections of cells of the nervous system, although walking becomes established before speech. In this function, too, man adjusts with more freedom to his surroundings than do some herd animals, for instance, who can walk, run, fall, and right themselves again within a few minutes of their birth regardless of the terrain on which the animal happens to be born. The functions established and fixed from birth show only small variations from one individual to another, while differences are the rule in the functions developed by the individual through his personal experience.

Dynamic aspects of posture

As long as we consider the standing and sitting postures as static conditions it is difficult to describe them in a way that might lead to improvement. If this is what we seek, we must examine their dynamic aspect. From the dynamic point of view, every stable posture is one of a series of positions that constitute a movement. In moving from side to side a pendulum passes through the position of stability at maximum speed. When the pendulum is in the stable state, at the midpoint of its path, it will remain there without moving until some outside force is applied to it. This stable position requires no energy for its maintenance. In walking, getting up, or sitting down, the human body of necessity from time to time also passes through the upright stable position that requires no energy. However, in cases where movements are not perfectly adjusted to gravity, the body's passage through the stable position is not clearly defined and the muscles continue to perform superfluous work.

No effort is required to maintain the standing and sitting postures, which are positions of stability. In the stable state only a minimum of energy is required for the beginning of any movement, and therefore none in order to remain at rest.

Automatic and voluntary control

Most of the theoretical and practical difficulties disappear when due consideration is paid to the fact that the voluntary muscles that respond to our intention will at the same time also react to orders from the other, unconscious parts of the nervous system. Under ordinary conditions automatic control takes over, although the voluntary control can come in at any desired moment. When the fastest possible reaction is needed, as when there is danger of falling or a sudden threat to life, then the automatic system will do all its work before we can even understand what is happening. We need only slip on a banana skin to discover that our body will in general right itself "by itself" in a reflex movement of which the voluntary control is not even aware.

We know if we are in the stable position through the kinesthetic sense of our muscles. If control over the muscles is with the voluntary system, then we are in the stable position; if it shifts to the automatic system and voluntary control ceases for a moment, the position is no longer stable. Voluntary control will return as soon as the automatic system has succeeded in bringing the body back to a stable position.

Origin of the distortion of sensations

Anything that tends to lessen the sensitivity of the power of discrimination will slow down response to stimuli. Posture will be adjusted only when its divergence from the stable position is already considerable, that is, when the adjustment has become more urgent and requires more muscular effort. This reduces even more precise awareness of the change; the entire system of action and control has taken on coarser dimensions. Ultimately there will be serious failure in control and even damage to the system.

One of the original causes of such a course of events is pain, which may have either a physical or an emotional origin. Pain that undermines confidence in the body and self is the main cause of deviations from the ideal posture. Pain of this kind reduces the individual's value in his own eyes. Nervous tension rises, which in turn reduces sensitivity once more; so we do not sense continued small deviations from the ideal position, and the muscles tense without the individual's even being aware of the effort he is making. Control may become so much distorted that while we think we are doing nothing we are in fact straining muscles needlessly.

Sensitivity in voluntary action

It seems reasonable to suppose that if we were to increase the degree of our awareness of muscular effort when our muscles are working as the result of voluntary action, then we shall also learn to recognize muscular efforts that, as the result of habit, are normally concealed from our conscious mind. If we can rid ourselves of such superfluous effort we shall recognize the ideal stable position with greater clarity. Then we shall have "returned" to the stage in which all conscious muscular effort to maintain equilibrium disappears, for this equilibrium is maintained solely by the older parts of the nervous system, which will find for us the best possible position compatible with the individual's inherited physical structure.

The dynamics of equilibrium

Let us return to the dynamic view of physical stability in order to learn from it as much as is possible. We saw that the stable position of the ordinary pendulum lies at the midpoint of its path, when the pull of gravity seeks to hold the pendulum in a purely vertical position. The force that first set the pendulum swinging is finally absorbed by friction, the movements becoming progressively smaller, until the pendulum remains at rest in the stable position; it can be moved by the application of a minimum of force applied in any direction other than the vertical. This is equally true for any body in a state of equilibrium. Thus, for instance, a tree that has grown upright will bend its top in whatever direction the wind is blowing. In the same way good upright posture is that from which a minimum muscular effort will move the body with equal ease in any desired direction. This means that in the upright position there must be no muscular effort deriving from voluntary control, regardless of whether this effort is known and deliberate or concealed from the consciousness by habit.

Swinging while standing

Stand and try to let your body swing lightly from side to side, as though it were a tree being bent by the wind. Pay attention to the movement of the spine and the head. Continue to make 10 to 15 small and quiet movements like this until you can observe a connection between these movements and your breathing. Then try similar movements backward and forward instead of sideways. You will soon observe that the movement backward is easier and larger, in most cases, than the forward movement, during which a certain amount of strian will be sensed in the ankles.

The points of strain vary with the individual. Only in rare cases will there be so perfect an organization of all the muscles of the chest—including those of the shoulders, the collarbone, the nape of the neck, the ribs, and the diaphragm—that you will be able to observe a continuous relationship between forward and backward movements and the process of breathing, as in the previous movements sideways.

Now move the body so that the top of the head marks a circle in a horizontal plane. Continue until you can feel that all the work is being done by the lower half of the legs and that all the movement can be felt in the ankles. Try swinging sideways again, and then backward and forward and in circles, in both directions, but this time let the weight of the body rest mainly on the right foot, while only the big toe of the left foot touches the floor. The left leg should take no part in the movement except to the extent that it helps the body to maintain its balance and makes it possible to carry out the movements accurately without interfering with breathing. Repeat these movements with most of the weight on the left foot. Repeat each of these movements 20 to 30 times until they can be carried out as smoothly and comfortably as possible.

Movement while sitting

Sit on the front edge of a chair. Place your feet on the floor, fairly far apart, and relax the muscles of the legs until the knees can be moved sideways and also forward in an easy movement from the ankles. In this position move the trunk from side to side until a light swinging movement is obtained that is coordinated with similarly smooth breathing. After a pause begin similar movements forward and backward until you become aware of movement in the hip joints and the pelvis, and of the backward and forward movement of the knees.

Now move the trunk in a circular path in such a way that the top of the head marks a circle, the head being supported on the spine as on a rod. There should be no changes in the relative positions of the vertebrae, the spine moving as though it were fastened to the chair at its lower end, near the coccyx, with the head balanced on its upper end; the head draws its circles as though the spine were the delimiting line of a cone standing on its point. Reverse the direction of the movement and continue until all hindrances to the movement disappear and it becomes continuous, fluid, and smooth.

The dynamic link between standing and sitting

We have now reached the most important point of all: the dynamic link between sitting and standing. Most people feel that the change from sitting to standing requires effort; without knowing it they gird themselves for this effort by contracting the muscles at the back of the neck, thereby drawing the head back and pointing the chin forward. This superfluous muscular effort stems from wanting to stiffen the chest for the effort to be made by the legs mainly in the extensors of the knees, the muscles that straighten the knees. We shall see this effort is also superfluous. All these movements indicate the intention to get up by means of a vigorous movement of the head, which draws the whole weight of the trunk behind it.

Concerning the voluntary control and the old reflex control, as we have called them, the interference consists of the fact that the feet press down on the floor in a voluntary movement before the body's center of gravity has moved forward over the soles of the feet. When the center of gravity has really moved forward over the feet a reflex movement will originate in the old nervous system and straighten the legs; this automatic movement will not be felt as an effort at all.

The conscious pressing on the floor with the feet usually takes place too soon, before the reflex stimulus is at its height. As voluntary control is overriding in slow movements, it is liable in this case to interfere with the primitive reflex control and prevent the movement from being carried out in the natural, organic, and efficient way. Our awareness must discern this organic need. Such discernment is perhaps the truest "knowledge of self."

The interference that develops is as follows: When the feet are pressed down too soon in the attempt to straighten the legs, the pelvis is held forcibly in place and its upper part may even be pushed back a little. Rising is attempted by the stomach muscles, which pull the head forward and down. But the body will fall back into a sitting position if the momentum of this movement is insufficient to raise the weight of the pelvis onto the legs, which are stiffened in an unyielding position and do not bend at the knee and ankle joints. Such failure to complete the movement may be observed among old or enfeebled persons who are not strong enough to carry out the superfluous efforts described above in addition to the effort actually needed to get up, although the latter is relatively small and within the capacity of even the old or weak.

Measure your mistakes and improvement

Place bathroom scales under your feet while sitting down before you begin the following exercise. Then get up in your accustomed manner. When you place your feet on the scales, you will observe that the needle will move to a point marking approximately a quarter of your weight as the weight of your legs. Stand up and watch the needle while you are doing so. The needle will swing far beyond the point marking your weight, return to a lower point, oscillate backward and forward, and finally come to rest at the right figure.

When you think that you have improved in getting up, check again with the scales. If the movement is now efficient you will find that the pointer moves gradually, parallel to your rising, and no longer swings past the correct figure for your weight. This shows that the movement no longer involves superfluous acceleration. If you try to calculate how much wasted effort you have now saved, you will also see how little effort is necessary to get up properly.

Now sit on the front edge of the chair again and let your body rock forward and backward in movements that continue to become larger but without any sudden increase in effort at any point.

Avoid all direct intention to get up, for this will result in the unnoticed return to your habitual manner of getting up. No effort greater than that involved in the rocking movement is actually required to get up. How is it done? Here are several aids that are all worth trying, even if you succeed with the first:

1. **Avoid conscious mobilization of the leg muscles.** During the forward movement think about lifting the knees and feet from the floor, so that the swing forward will not make you contract the muscles of the thigh, whose function is to straighten the legs. The contraction of these muscles results in increased pressure of the feet on the floor. The pelvis will now leave the chair without any additional effort and the sitting position will change into the standing position.

2. **Avoid conscious mobilization of the neck muscles.** During the swinging backward and forward catch hair at the top of your head and pull it gently in line with the cervical spine so lightly that you can feel whether the neck muscles are being tensed. When there is no tensing of the nape muscles in the forward swing, there is no sudden extra pressure through the feet, and the movement forward will—after a few attempts—bring the body into the standing position without any change in breathing, that is, without any superfluous effort by the chest.

Repeat this exercise using the left hand to hold the hair on the head. There is usually a difference in effect between the two hands.

3. **Cease intention to get up.** The movement forward should be continued to the point at which an effort is felt in the legs and breathing apparatus, that is, the point at which the rhythmical movement is arrested and muscular effort increases. At this point rising is no longer a continuation of the previous movement but a sudden jerking effort. Stop all further movement and remain frozen in the position in which the swinging movement ceased. Halt the intention to get up and see which part of the body relaxes

as a result. This is the effort that was superfluous to correct getting up. This is not easy, and you will have to pay close attention to detect it. If you stop the intention to rise, the frozen position immediately becomes as comfortable as sitting down, and it becomes equally easy to complete the movement into the upright position or to sit down again.

4. **Rhythmical knee movements.** Sit on the edge of a chair, place your feet on the ground comfortably, far apart. Now start moving your knees together and apart several times, until the movement becomes rhythmical, regular, and easy. Catch the hair at the top of your head and bring yourself into a standing position without any interruption in the movement of your knees. If the body is not properly organized the movement of the knees will falter, if only for a moment, or else you will try to get up at the exact moment when the knees are at one of the end positions of their movement, either farthest apart or close together. In either of these positions the knees can cease their movement without its being noticeable.

5. **Separating action from intention.** One of the requirements of improved action is to separate action from intention, as in the following exercise, which is both an aid to learning and a means to test the quality of the action performed.

Sit on a chair as before, with the back of another chair in front of you. Rest your hands on the back of the chair in front and, instead of thinking about getting up, think about raising your seat and at the same time get up. While you are standing, place your hands on the back of the chair in front of you and, instead of thinking about sitting down, think that you will lower your seat back onto the chair, and complete the movement with this in your mind.

Placing your seat on the chair is a means of sitting down, just as raising it is a means of getting up. In this way your attention is focused on the means by which the action is performed, not on the intention of performing it. Many people are able to rise or sit down in this fashion without thinking about what they are doing. The action is properly carried out when it makes no difference whether the performer thinks about the intention or about the means of carrying it out. When the action is faulty an observer can tell at once which of the two modes of thought the performer was following during the movement.

Concentration on the aim may cause excessive tension

It is easy to shift your attention from the aim of a simple action to the means of its performance and to carry out the latter. In a complicated action, the greater the desire to achieve its aim, the greater will be the difference in its performance according to which of the two modes of thinking are adopted.

A too-strong wish for the aim often causes internal tension. This tension not only hinders your achieving the desired aim, but may even endanger life—as, for instance, in crossing a road, when the aim is at all costs to catch a bus on the other side and attention is diverted completely from the surroundings.

Performance is improved by the separation of the aim from the means

In most cases where an action is linked to a strong desire, the efficiency of the action may be improved by separating the aim from the means of achieving it. A motorist in a desperate hurry to reach his destination, for instance, will fare better if he entrusts the wheel to a man who is a good driver but not desperate to reach the destination in time.

Serious obstacles to performance may occur when both the action and the achievement of the aim depend on the old section of the nervous system—old in the evolutionary sense—over which our control is involuntary. These actions might include sex, falling asleep, or evacuation of the bowels. The action may be performed as if the aim were the means, and sometimes as though the means were the aim. It is therefore good to study this problem when both the aim and the means are simple in order to apply the understanding so gained to more important actions.

Efficient force acts in the direction of the movement

Sit on the edge of a chair and place the tips of the fingers of your right hand on the top of your head. The contact should be light enough to make it possible to detect changes in tension in the nape of the neck. Raise and lower your chin (by moving the muscles of the nape and neck) and observe whether your fingertips record the movement of the head.

Increase the movement of your head forward and upward by moving your hip joints until your seat rises from the chair and you are standing, but without a sudden increase of effort in the legs at any stage of the movement.

You will see that control of the movement by the fingertips and the smooth upward action to standing have organized the chest muscles so that the ribs and chest hang from the spine and are not stiffened by the muscles.

For the weight of the chest to be taken by the spine and for breathing to be free during the entire movement, the effort made by the muscles of the hip joints must be so directed that the resultant force will go through the spine itself. No parasitic forces should develop that will cause a change in the angle of the head and the neck vertebrae or induce curvature in the spine.

Before this movement can become precise and effective, practice must increase the feeling of ease and power until you no longer try to brace yourself for the effort by holding your breath or tensing your chest. The tendency to hold one's breath is instinctive, part of an attempt to prevent the establishment of shearing stresses or forces likely to shift the vertebrae horizontally, out of the vertical alignment of the spinal column that they constitute.

Lack of choice makes strain habitual

As long as superfluous effort is invested in any action, man must throw up defenses, must brace himself to great effort that is neither comfortable, pleasurable, nor desirable. The lack of choice of whether to make an effort or not turns an action into habit, and in the end nothing appears more natural than that to which he is accustomed, even if it is opposed to all reason or necessity.

Habit makes it easier to persist in an action, and for this reason it is extremely valuable in general. Nevertheless we easily over indulge in habits until self-criticism is silenced and our ability to discern is diminished, which gradually turns us into machines that act without thinking.

Effective action improves the body and its capacity to act

The effectiveness of an action is judged first of all by the simple standard of whether it achieves its purpose. But that test is not sufficient. Action must also improve a living and developing body at least to the extent that the same action will be carried out more effectively the next time. For instance, it is possible to tighten a screw with a kitchen knife, but both the knife and the screw will be damaged. The human body is capable of so many different types of movement and action that it is difficult to define briefly which movements are effective, and every definition is bound to be oversimplified. Nevertheless we shall try to clarify what makes for a well-performed action.

Reversibility is the mark of voluntary movement

If we simply move the hand from right to left and back again, at medium speed, we shall all agree that the movement is satisfactory if it is possible to interrupt and reverse it at any point, to continue it again in the original direction, or to decide to make some altogether different movement instead.

This quality is inherent in the simple type of movement described above even if we do not know it, and it is found in all fully conscious, deliberate movements; we shall refer to it as reversibility. A tap on the sinew just below the kneecap produces a jerk in the leg that is entirely a reflex, a movement that we cannot arrest, reverse, or change. The same applies to clonic movements, shivering, or spasms. None of these are reversible because they are involuntary.

Light and easy movements are good

When we considered ways of getting up from a chair, we saw that a good deliberate movement is produced when there is no conflict between voluntary control and the body's automatic reaction to gravity, when the two combine and aid each other to perform an action that appears to have been directed by a single center. Voluntary control is usually effective with relatively slow movements, so long as the movement does not endanger the body or cause such pain that the automatic reaction takes over or bypasses the willed decision.

We saw also that the simple movement of the hand was good without any prior knowledge of what constitutes good movement. Light and easy movements are good ones, as a rule.

It is important to learn how to turn strenuous movements into good ones—that is, into movements that are first of all effective but also smooth and easy.

Avoiding difficulties establishes behavioral norms

As a general rule, human beings cease to develop or to improve their ability to adjust to circumstances at about thirteen or fourteen years of age. Activities of the brain, emotions, and body that are still difficult or impossible at this age will remain permanently beyond the bounds of the habitual. The result is that man remains far more limited in his capacities than he need be.

These limitations usually impose themselves upon the individual as a result of difficulties encountered in the process of physiological or social development. When the individual repeatedly experiences a certain difficulty, he usually abandons the activity that he has found hard to master, at which he has not succeeded, or that has proved disagreeable in some way. He establishes a rule for himself, saying, for instance, "I cannot learn how to dance," or "I am not sociable by nature," or "I shall never understand mathematics." The limits that he thus sets for himself will stop his development not only in the fields that he has decided to abandon, but also in other areas; they may even influence his entire personality.

The feeling that something is "too difficult" will spread and engulf other activities. It is difficult to estimate the importance to the individual of the qualities he lacks and of the things he therefore never tries, and thus the losses he incurs without knowing it are incalculable.

There is no limit to improvement

The man who was used to reading by the light of a torch or of an oil lamp felt the wax candle to be the ultimate improvement and paid no attention to the smoke, soot, and smell it gave off. When we consider the further development of artificial light we see that the limits we set to it are dictated only by our ignorance. Every time that we expand the limits of our knowledge, our sensibility and the precision of our actions increase and the limits of what is considered natural and normal also expand.

The more an individual advances his development the greater will be his ease of action, the ease synonymous with harmonious organization of the senses and the muscles. When activity is freed of tension and superfluous effort the resulting ease makes for greater sensitivity and better discrimination, which make for still greater ease in action. He will now be able to identify unnecessary effort even in actions that formerly seemed easy to him. As this sensitivity in action is further refined, it continues to become increasingly delicate up to a certain level. In order to pass this limit there must be improved organization of the entire personality. But at this stage further advance will no longer be achieved slowly and gradually, but by a sudden step. Ease of action is developed to the point where it becomes a new quality with new horizons.

Suppose that an actor, speaker, or teacher who has suffered from hoarseness begins to study ways of improving his enunciation in order to rid himself of his trouble. He will start by trying to locate the excess effort he makes in his breathing apparatus and throat. When he has learned to reduce the expenditure of effort and to speak more easily, he will note to his surprise that he has also been doing unnecessary work with the muscles of his jaw and tongue, work of which he was previously unaware and which contributed to his hoarseness. Thus the ease achieved in one area will make closer and more accurate observation possible in related areas.

When he continues to practice his new achievements and can use the muscles of his tongue and jaw without effort, he may discover that he has been using only the back of his mouth and his throat to produce his voice, not the front part of his mouth. This involved a greater effort in breathing because greater air pressure was needed to force the voice through the mouth. When he learns to use the front of his mouth as well, speaking will have become far easier, and he will discover that there has also been improvement in the use of the muscles of the chest and diaphragm.

He will now discover to his surprise that the interference with the muscles of the chest, diaphragm, and front of the mouth were due to continuous tension in the muscles of the nape of the neck that forced his head and chin forward and distorted his breathing and speaking organs. This will lead him to further discoveries connected with his manner of standing and of moving.

What all this means is that the total personality is involved in proper speech. But even these discoveries, the improvements that they brought about, and the ease of action that resulted are still not the whole story. The man discovers that his voice, previously limited to a single octave, will now reach both considerably higher and lower pitches. He discovers an entirely new quality in his voice and finds that he can sing. This again opens up new possibilities in wider fields and reveals capacities of which he had never dreamed before.

Use large muscles for the heavy work

For effective movement the heavy work of moving the body must be shifted to the muscles designed for this purpose.

If we look carefully we will see that the largest and strongest muscles are connected to the pelvis. Most of the work is done by these muscles, particularly the buttocks, thighs, and the abdominals. As we move away from the center of the body to the limbs the muscles gradually become more slender. The muscles of the limbs are intended to direct their movements accurately, while the main power of the pelvic muscles is conducted through the bones of the limbs to the point at which it is required to operate.

In a well-organized body work done by the large muscles is passed on to its final destination through the bones by weaker muscles, but without losing much of its power on the way.

Forces working at an angle to the main path cause damage

Under ideal conditions the work done by the body passes lengthwise through the spine and the bones of the limbs, that is, in something as near to a straight line as possible. If the body forms angles to the main line of action, part of the effort made by the pelvic muscles will not reach the point at which it was directed; in addition, ligaments and joints will suffer damage. If, for instance, we push against something with one hand with the arm fully extended, the force of the pelvic muscles will operate straight through the arm and hand. If, however, the arm is bent at a right angle at the elbow, the force in the hand itself cannot be larger than that of the forearm alone. Action becomes difficult and uncomfortable because the force of the large muscles cannot be helpful since it is almost wholly absorbed by the body.

When the force of the large pelvic muscles fails to be transmitted by the skeletal structure through the bones, it becomes difficult to refrain from stiffening the chest in order to permit the directional muscles to perform at least a part of the work that should be done with ease by the pelvic muscles. Good bodily organization makes it possible to carry out most normal actions without any feeling of effort or strain.

Develop paths of ideal action

The ideal path of action for the skeleton as it moves from one position to another—say, from sitting to standing or from lying to sitting—is the path through which it would move if it had no muscles at all, if the bones were linked only by ligaments. In order to get up from the floor by the shortest and most efficient path, the body must be organized in such a way that the bones will follow the path indicated by a skeleton pulled up by its head. If they follow this path the muscular effort will be transmitted through the bones and all the effort of the pelvic muscles will be turned into useful work.

Lesson 3

Some Fundamental Properties of Movement

In this lesson you will learn to recognize some of the fundamental properties of the control mechanisms of the voluntary muscles. You will find that about thirty slow, light, and short movements are sufficient to change the fundamental tonus of the muscles, that is, the state of their contraction before their activation by the will. Once the change of tonus is effected, it will spread to the entire half of the body containing the part originally worked on. An action becomes easy to perform and the movement becomes light when the huge muscles of the center of the body do the bulk of the work and the limbs only direct the bones to the destination of the effort.

Scan the state of your body

Lie down on your back. Place your legs a comfortable distance apart. Stretch your arms out above your head, slightly apart, so that the left arm will be approximately in a straight line with the right leg and the right arm in line with the left leg.

Close your eyes and try to check the areas of the body that are in contact with the floor. Pay attention to the manner in which the heels lie on the floor, whether the pressure upon them is equal,

91

and whether the point of contact is at exactly the same points at both heels. In the same way examine the contact made with the floor by the calf muscles, the back of the knees, the hip joints, the floating ribs, the upper ribs, and the shoulder blades. Pay attention to the respective distances between the shoulders, elbows, wrists and the floor.

A few minutes of study will show that there is a considerable difference between the two sides of the body at the shoulders, elbows, ribs, and so forth. Many people will find that in this position their elbows do not touch the floor at all but are suspended in space. The arms do not rest on the ground, and it becomes difficult to maintain them in this position until the examination is over.

Discover the latent work of the muscles

We have a coccyx, five lumbar, twelve dorsal, and seven cervical vertebrae. On which vertebrae in the pelvic region is pressure heaviest? Do all the lumbar vertebrae (girdle) touch the floor? If not, what is raising them above the floor? On which of the dorsal or back vertebrae is pressure heaviest? At the beginning of this lesson most people will find that two or three of the vertebrae make clear contact with the floor while the others form arches between them. This is surprising, because our intention was to lie at rest on the floor, without making any effort or movement, so that in theory each of the vertebrae and ribs should sink to the floor and touch it at least at one point. A skeleton without muscles would indeed lie in this way. It seems, therefore, that the muscles raise the parts of the body to which they are attached without our being conscious of it.

It is impossible to stretch out the entire spine on the floor without a conscious strain upon several sections. As soon as this conscious effort is once more relaxed, the sections affected will again move up and away from the floor. In order to settle the whole of the spine on the floor we must stop the work the muscles are doing without our knowledge. How can we do this if deliberate and conscious effort is not successful? We shall have to try an indirect method.

A new start for each movement

Lie down once more and stretch out your arms and legs as before. Probably at least the backs of your hands will now touch the floor, and perhaps also your elbows and upper arms. Now raise your right upper arm, by a shoulder movement only, until the back of the hand just ceases touching the floor, making, in fact, a slow, infinitely small movement. Then let the arm drop back to the floor and rest there. Raise the arm again until the back of the hand leaves the floor. Repeat this twenty or twenty-five times. Each time you have raised and lowered the arm make a complete pause, stop all movement, and let the next movement be an entirely new and separate action.

Coordinating breathing and movement

If you pay close attention you will feel that the back of your hand is beginning to creep along the floor a little as the arm stretches before it is raised. When the movement has been repeated a number of times you will find that it is becoming coordinated with the breathing rhythm. The raising and lengthening of the arm will be found to coincide accurately with the moment at which air begins to be expelled from the lungs.

Pause and observe

At the end of twenty-five movements bring the arms slowly down to the sides of the body. Make sure that this movement is carried out in stages, as a quick movement is likely to cause pain in the shoulder that has been working. Draw up your knees into a bent position and rest for a moment. While you are resting observe the difference you can now feel between the right and left sides of your body.

Slow and gradual movement

Now turn and lie on your stomach, with arms and legs spread out as before. Raise your right elbow slowly from the shoulder until it leaves the floor (now the hand will not necessarily lift as well) and then let the elbow sink down again.

In order to carry out this movement as described the arms must be stretched out comfortably above the head, that is, in such a way that the distance between the hands is smaller than that between the elbows, with the latter slightly bent.

Continue to raise the elbow just as you begin to expel the air from your lungs. Repeat this at least twenty times. If the movement is slow and gradual, as it should be, you will discover that the elbow is now "creeping" with the arm, that is, it stretches a little before it begins to leave the floor. As the elbow begins to lift sufficiently to draw the wrist after it the hand will also begin to leave the floor.

Eliminate superfluous effort

When a man lifts his wrist in this position it is rare for the hand itself to remain hanging down relaxed. Most people unknowingly tense the extensors (the muscles of the outer side of the forearm) of the hand and the hand is raised so that an angle is formed between the back of the hand and the forearm. Gradually, by paying attention, it is possible to cease this superfluous and unintentional muscular effort.

To do this, we must relax the muscles of the forearm, not only those of the fingers. When the relaxation is complete the hand will drop down and an angle will be formed between the palm and the inner side of the forearm. If the elbow is then raised, the hand will hang down relaxed.

Use the muscles of the back

Continue this movement and lift the whole arm, with the elbow and hand, until you feel that no muscular effort is needed any longer to do so and the only effort comes from the shoulder region. To make it easier for the shoulders to rise from the floor you will have to bring the muscles of the back into action. The shoulder will then come up and away from the floor together with the shoulder blade and the right upper side of the chest.

Lie on your back again and rest, and observe the difference in the way your shoulders, chest, and arms now make contact with the floor on the right and left sides.

Simultaneous action

Stretch out your arms above your head again, hands apart. Stretch out your legs, feet apart. Very, very slowly, simultaneously raise your right leg and your right arm. Only a small movement is needed, just enough to lift the back of your hand and your heel free of the floor. Pay attention to see whether your hand and heel return to the floor absolutely together, or one after the other. When you decide which of them reaches the ground first, you will discover that this limb also rises off the ground ahead of the other. It is not easy to achieve absolutely simultaneous action in this movement. Generally a small discrepancy will remain between the movement of arm and leg.

In order to achieve a degree of accuracy raise the arm just as you begin to expel the air from your lungs. Then raise your leg as you begin to breathe out. Finally, move both arm and leg as you breathe out. This will improve coordination between the two limbs.

Sensing lengthening in the spine

Now raise the arm and leg alternately. Watch to see whether the lumbar vertebrae rise a little from the floor when the leg is raised alone, without the arm, and whether the movement of these vertebrae is affected at all when the arm is raised together with the leg.

The lumbar vertebrae rise from the floor because the leg is lifted by muscles attached to the front of the pelvis. The muscles of the back are also involved in raising these vertebrae. Is the work done by these back muscles necessary or superfluous?

Turn the leg to the right, that is, turn the hip joint, knee, and foot to the right. Now, very, very slowly, lift the leg in this position and observe how the changed position of the leg affects the movement of the hip vertebrae. It will gradually become clear that if leg and arm are raised simultaneously, at the moment when air begins to be expelled from the lungs, then the work is being done by the muscles of stomach and chest in coordination. The lumbar vertebrae no longer rise but are, on the contrary, pressed against the floor. The raising of arm and leg becomes easier and there is a feeling as though the body were being lengthened in the process. This feeling of the spine lengthening accompanies most actions of the body when they are properly carried out.

Superfluous efforts shorten the body

In almost every case excess tension remaining in the muscles causes the spine to be shortened. Unnecessary effort accompanying an action tends to shorten the body. In every action in which a degree of difficulty is anticipated the body is drawn together as a protective device against this difficulty. It is precisely this reinforcement of the body that requires the unnecessary effort and prevents the body from organizing itself correctly for action. The limit of ability must be widened by means of study and understanding rather than by stubborn effort and attempts to protect the body.

Further, this self-protection and superfluous effort in action are an expression of the individual's lack of self-confidence. As soon as a person is conscious that he is placing a strain on his powers he makes a greater effort of the will to reinforce his body for the action, but in fact he is forcing superfluous effort on himself. The act resulting from this attempt to reinforce the body will never be either graceful or stimulating, and will arouse no wish in the individual to repeat it. While it is possible to reach the desired aim in this tortuous fashion, the price paid for its achievement is higher than appears at first sight.

Rest for a minute and observe the change that has taken place in the contact made by the pelvis with the floor as well as the difference between the left and the right sides of the body.

What is more comfortable?

Roll over onto your stomach and stretch your arms out above your head, wide apart. Spread your legs and slowly raise your right arm and right leg together. Observe the position of your head when you are about to raise your limbs. Does it face to the right or the left, is it lying on the floor? Try to raise your arm and leg as you breathe out. Do this several times, first with your right cheek resting on the floor, that is, facing to the left. Then repeat with your forehead resting on the floor, and finally with the left cheek on the floor.

Now compare the amount of effort required in the three positions, and decide in which position the movement is easiest to carry out. In a more or less well-organized body the most comfortable position will have the left cheek on the floor. Repeat the movement about twenty-five times and note how it becomes gradually clearer that the pressure of the body on the floor shifts to the left side of the stomach, between the chest and the pelvis.

Remain on your stomach and continue to raise your right arm

and leg as before, but now, with each movement, also raise your head, letting your eyes follow the movement of the hand. Turn onto your back and rest after twenty-five movements. Then repeat the movement as before, raising arm, leg, and head together. Observe how differently the body is lying on the floor compared to before the exercise. Identify separately the areas of the body and of the floor that are now in contact. Note the exact point where the pressure is greatest. Repeat the movement twenty-five times and then stop.

Which eye is open wider?

Get up, walk about a little, check the difference in sensation in the right and left sides of the body, the difference in the apparent weight and length of the arms, and the difference in the length of the legs. Examine your face: Look in a mirror to see that one side of your face looks fresher, folds and wrinkles on that side are less marked, and one eye is open wider than the other. Which eye is it?

Try to recall whether you noticed at the checks carried out earlier after each series of movements that one arm and one leg became progressively longer than the limbs on the other side of the body. Do not try to overcome the sensation of difference between the two sides of the body but allow it to persist and continue to observe it until it lessens and finally disappears. If no disturbance is encountered that interrupts attention, such as annoyance or a high degree of tension, then the difference should remain noticeable for many hours, or at least several. During this period observe which side of your body functions better and on which sides movements are carried out more smoothly.

Work on the left side

Repeat all the movements detailed thus far in this lesson, but with the left side of your body.

Diagonal movement

When you have finished the movements using the left side of your body, raise your right arm and left leg together very, very slowly, and repeat twenty-five times. Observe the changes in the relative positions of the vertebrae and ribs, and note that the parts of the back on which the body is resting are quite different to those identified after the limbs on one side of the body were raised together.

After a short rest raise the left arm and the right leg together twenty-five times, and then rest. Now raise all four limbs and the head together as the air is expelled from the lungs. Repeat this movement twenty-five times. After a rest, raise only the four limbs, leaving the head resting on the floor.

Repeat these combinations of movements lying on your stomach.

Finally, lie on your back and observe all the areas now in contact with the floor, starting with the heels right up to the head, as you did at the beginning of the lesson. Note the changes that have taken place, particularly along the spine.

Lesson 4

Differentiation
of Parts
and Functions
in Breathing

Now you will learn to recognize the movements of the ribs, dia-phragm, and abdomen that make up your breathing. Proper adjustment of these movements is necessary in order to breathe deeply and easily. You will be able to recognize the difference in the length of the periods of breathing in and out, and to realize that the process of breathing adjusts itself to the posture of the body with respect to gravity. The lower ribs move more than the upper ones and contribute more to breathing. You will finally see that breathing becomes easier and more rhythmical when the body is held erect without any conscious effort, that is, when its entire weight is supported by the skeletal structure.

Volume of the chest and breathing

Lie on your back; stretch out your legs, feet apart, and draw up your knees. The soles of your feet will now be resting on the ground as in the standing position, with feet apart. Move your knees together and apart several times until each knee is poised in the plane passing through its own foot on a line drawn through the center of the heel and between each big toe and that next to it. No muscular effort is required to maintain the knees in this position.

Draw in air to fill your lungs, increasing the volume of your chest as far as you can without discomfort. Many people breathe without letting their breastbone move relative to the spine. Instead of increasing the volume of their chest in accordance with its structure, they hollow their back, that is to say raise the entire chest from the ground, including the lower part of the back, so that its interior volume is increased only by the movement of the floating ribs.

See whether your spine presses on the ground for the entire length of the chest as the latter expands and the breastbone moves away from the spine. Do not attempt to force the spine down; make no effort. Simply fill the lungs with air, watch for the chest to rise, and see whether the spine is pressed against the floor at the same time.

Stop the movement. Wait until you need to breathe, and try again. Repeat this a number of times.

Breathing movements without breathing

When you have done this and the movement has become clear, try to raise the chest as before, but without breathing in. That is, make the breathing movements with the chest, but without either drawing in or expelling air. Repeat this several times, until you again feel the need to breathe. Fill your lungs and repeat the movements of the chest. Stop and rest, and after five or six repetitions of this series of movements check your breathing. In what way has it changed since before you began the exercise?

Increasing the volume of the lower abdomen

Place your fingertips on your abdomen with your elbows on the floor. Wait until your lungs are filled with air. Compress your chest as though to expel the air, but hold your breath—don't breathe out. The increasing pressure of air will raise the pressure in the abdomen, which can be directed downward in the direction of the anal ring. As the air is forced down below the navel, the lower part of the stomach will become round as a football.

Notice that your hands will rise and move away from your sides as your stomach swells.

In the quasic liquid contents of the abdomen pressure distributes itself equally in all directions. However, most people at first fail to expand their stomach in all directions in this exercise unless they have a strong and well-developed back and hips. Instead, they strain the muscles of the back in the neighborhood of the hips until the spine rises from the ground at the hips. Attention must therefore be paid to establishing equal pressure in the stomach in all directions, including backward, toward the floor. When you can do this you will find that pushing the stomach out or forward will expel the air from the lungs. Wait until the lungs fill up once more, and then expel the air by pushing the stomach forward and expanding it all round until you can feel the fleshy parts around the hips pressing against the floor. Rest and observe the changes that have taken place in the quality of the breathing movement.

Seesaw movements of the diaphragm

Fill your lungs with air and hold your breath—do not breathe either in or out; then similarly contract the chest and expand the stomach in sequential movements. Now expand the chest and pull the stomach in again, and repeat these alternate movements as long as you can without breathing either in or out. It is quite easy to carry out five or six such alternating movements of the chest and stomach as though they were the two sides of a balance, with one side going up as the other goes down.

Repeat the whole exercise five or six times. Then try it again, but as fast as possible without discomfort. When the alternate movements of stomach and chest are carried out fast enough it will be possible to distinguish a movement, and even a gargling sound, somewhere between the ribs and the navel. Something is changing its position there and pressing alternately upward, in the direction of the head, and downward, in the direction of the feet. This is the movement of the diaphragm. We are not normally aware of the diaphragm, but in this exercise we can indirectly identify its position in the body without knowing its actual anatomical location.

Normal breathing

Lie on your back; stretch out your arms and legs, feet apart. Repeat the alternate movements of the chest and stomach without changing your ordinary breathing rhythm. It is possible to carry out the alternate up-and-down movements of the chest and stomach while breathing normally, just as they can be carried out while holding your breath. In this way one may distinguish between movements that are essential to breathing and the superfluous movements that accompany it.

Repeat the movement twenty-five times. After resting for a minute turn onto your stomach, stretch your arms above your head, hands apart, and stretch out your legs, feet also apart, and continue the previous movement.

A truly symmetrical spine does not exist

It is rare to find a truly symmetrical spine. In most cases the plane of the shoulders and chest is twisted relative to the plane of the pelvis, and as a result, all movements are performed more easily on one side of the body than on the other. In the early years, when a child tends to make random movements of great variety, this does not matter at all. In maturity, however, persons tend to repeat a limited number of movements—sometimes for hours on end—to the neglect of other movements. The body then tends to accustom itself to this restricted number of movements, the skeletal structure adjusts to them, changes result, and posture becomes crooked.

Sensing the middle

It is important to observe whether the chest, when it is pushed out, first touches the ground exactly in the middle of the breastbone, and whether the stomach, in turn, touches the ground in the middle. This is not easy, for our powers of identifying such matters are insufficiently developed. A person may believe that his body is resting on the ground symmetrically, while an observer can see clearly that this is not the case. Nevertheless try this several times.

Now continue the exercise, but when you push out the chest let the left side press more clearly on the ground, and when you push out the stomach let its right side touch the ground first.

The whole back will now move obliquely from the right hip joint in the direction of the left shoulder. After twenty-five such movements repeat the previous exercise, trying to place the middle of the chest and stomach on the ground and observe the change that has taken place in the sensation of where this middle is located. Now do another twenty-five movements in the opposite way, resting the left side of the stomach and the right side of the chest on the ground. When you have done this, again try to rest the middle of chest and stomach on the ground at each movement and observe how clearly the middle can now be identified.

Roll onto your back. Repeat the alternating stomach and chest movements and notice how the chest movement has increased. Observe the sensation of free movement and try to identify the sections of your back where movement has become easier and is causing the sensation of release from constriction.

Seesaw movements lying on your side

Lie on your right side. Stretch out your right arm above your head and rest your head on the arm. Catch hold of your head with your left hand, with the fingers on the right temple, and the palm of the hand on the top of the head. Now raise your head with the help of the left hand until the left ear comes close to the left shoulder. With the head in this raised position, expand the chest in all directions and draw in the stomach; then compress the chest and expand the stomach, and observe the movements of the ribs on both sides. On the right side the floor will prevent any expansion of the ribs and the chest can now expand only on the left side, where the spreading apart of the ribs will force the head back somewhat toward the right arm.

Repeat this movement twenty-five times, then lie on your back and try to observe which parts of your back have sunk down and are now more clearly in contact with the floor.

Repeat, doing another twenty-five similar movements while lying on your left side.

Seesaw movements on the back

Lie on your back, raise your shoulders off the ground, and support yourself on both hands and forearms placed parallel to your body. Your chest will now be at an angle to the floor, and your head and shoulders free. Lower your head until the chin touches the breastbone. In this position once more make twenty-five seesaw movements of chest and stomach. Lie on your back to rest.

Raise yourself as before on elbows, forearms, and hands, but this time let your head drop back in the direction of the floor with the chin as far as possible from the breastbone. Make twenty-five alternating movements of stomach and chest; while doing this observe the movement of the spine.

Lie on your back and observe your breathing. There should by now be a clearly discernible improvement in your breathing, which will be easier and deeper.

Seesaw movements while kneeling

Kneel with your knees wide apart and your feet stretched out in a straight line with the lower leg (your toenails will be facing the floor). Now lower your head until its top touches the ground in front of you. Place your hands, palms down, on either side of your head to support part of your weight and protect your head against excessive pressure.

Fill your chest with air, draw in your stomach, then compress your chest while expanding the stomach again; repeat twenty-five times. While carrying out this exercise observe that when the chest is expanded the body moves forward in the direction of the head, and the head itself rolls forward a little on the ground. The chin moves back toward the breastbone and the muscles of the nape and back stretch and tighten while the spine curves a little higher. When the stomach is pushed out, on the other hand, the pelvis settles down and back as though you were about to sit on your heels. The back is less curved and the pelvic vertebrae form a concave line.

Repeat twenty-five times; lie on your back and observe the differences in breathing and in the contact of the back with the floor.

How the seesaw movement affects breathing

The effect on breathing will be greater this time than before. In the upright position the lungs and other breathing apparatus are suspended and pulled down to the lowest possible position by their weight. When air is breathed in, an active lifting effort is required in order to allow the lungs to expand. In the last exercise, in which the top of the head rested on the ground, the weight of the lung pulled it toward the head. Breathing in involved no lifting effort, but when breathing out some work had to be performed to raise the lung back to its deflated position. It should be remembered, also, that there are no muscles in the lung tissue itself, and the work of moving the lungs is done by the muscles of the ribs, diaphragm, and stomach.

Have you ever observed that in our usual upright position air is inhaled rapidly and expelled slowly? When we are speaking, for instance, there is scarcely any pause between one sentence and the next. We speak during the prolonged breathing out process that operates the vocal cords. With the top of our head resting on the ground, the exhaling process is short and rapid and inhaling is prolonged. Try to check this through your own experience.

Curvature of the spine and pelvic movement

Kneel with your knees apart. Lean on your head and hands as before. Move your left knee a little closer to your head. Repeat the seesaw movement of chest and stomach. When the chest is expanded the body will move forward toward the head roughly as before, but when the stomach is pushed out and the pelvis moves back into a sitting position, it will move only in the direction of the right heel, and the hips will twist out of alignment with the shoulders. Two different movements of the spine can now be observed: convex and concave curvature as before, and also a movement of the pelvis to the right and left with respect to the shoulders.

When you have completed twenty-five of these movements, lie on your back, rest, and observe changes in the chest, in your breathing, and in the contact of your back with the floor.

Now kneel again and make another twenty-five movements of the chest and stomach with your right knee closer to your head than your left. Observe the difference between the pelvic movement in this position and in the previous one. Try to discover the main cause of this difference. If you cannot find it now, you will learn to do so in time, when your ability to observe and distinguish movements has improved.

Widening your back [Ill. 1]

Sit on the floor with your knees far enough apart to allow you to place your feet together in the middle, resting on their outside edges, and with the soles touching. Place your right hand on the left side of your chest, on the lower ribs, and the left hand on the lower ribs of the right side, hugging your back. Lower your head, push out your chest, and draw in your stomach; reverse your breathing; and keep repeating these actions.

Observe the expansion of the ribs on your back, under your fingers. The chest does not expand in front because a part of its muscles is engaged in the movement of hugging your back. This time the lungs have expanded mainly as a result of the spreading of the lower back ribs. This is the most efficient breathing movement because it takes place at the point where the lungs are widest.

Make twenty-five such movements. Observe your back ribs; are they continuing to move?

Stand up. Observe whether your body is more erect than it was before the exercise. Feel the set of your shoulders, which should show a considerable difference. Check your breathing. It will undoubtedly be better than usual. This improvement is a step in the desired direction as the result of practical work. You cannot achieve such breathing by merely understanding the mechanism of breathing intellectually.

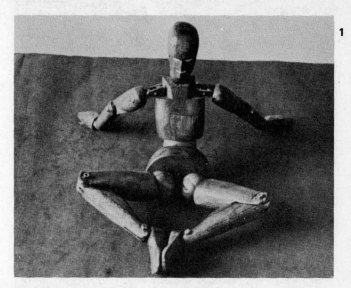

Sit on the floor . . . lean on both hands behind you . . . knees apart sideways . . . the soles of the feet against one another.

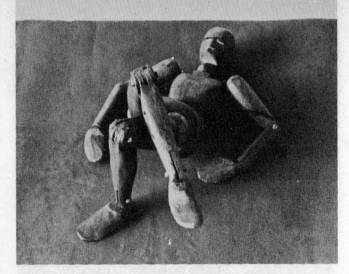

Lie on your back. Draw up your knees. Cross your right leg over the left knee.

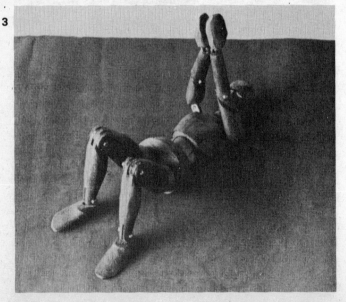

Come to the initial position . . . both feet on the floor . . . comfortably spread. Raise both arms . . . touch both palms, as if clapping . . . arms are straight up in the air with straight elbows.

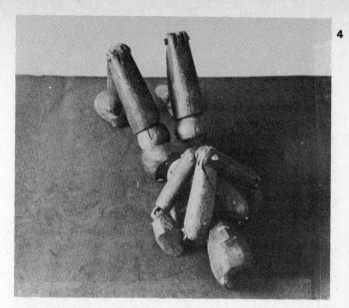

4

Lift left arm and put right arm underneath left armpit. Get hold of the left shoulder blade.

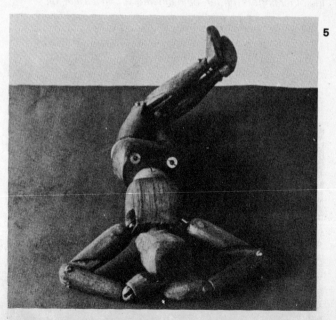

5

. . . knees bent at right angle . . . soles of the feet in the direction of the ceiling . . . imagine your ankles . . . and knees are tied together with a piece of string . . . tilt both legs.

6

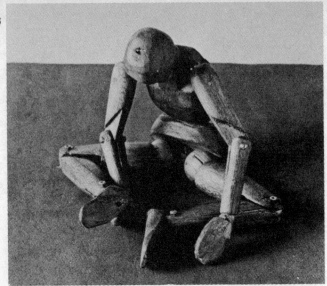

*Open your knees sideways . . . feet lie on their outer edges . . .
your right hand, palm turned upwards . . . the fingertips come
underneath the right heel . . . the thumb goes, [together] with all
the other fingers, underneath the heel . . . lift it a little bit.*

7

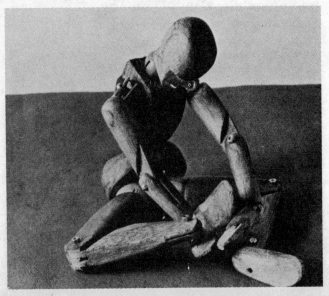

*. . . grip the toes . . . with the left hand, so that the small toe
rests in your left palm.*

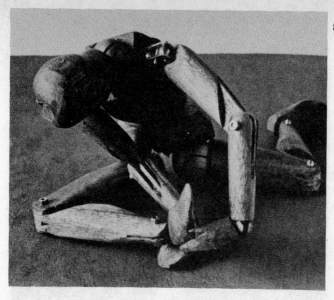

8

Sit up again . . . slightly move your body to the right, so that you can lean against the floor with your right knee and leg . . . left foot must move out of the way, to your left and maybe even backward . . . Then rock your head a little bit more to the right, over the knee.

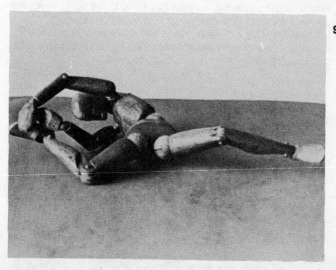

. . . your head a little bit more to the right, over the knee . . . near to the floor . . . you will suddenly find yourself rolling . . . roll over your right shoulder blade, with the left leg into the air and, probably, the left one leaving the floor too.

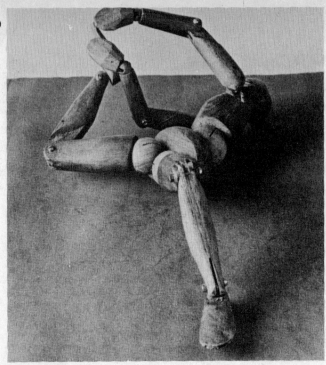

From the lying position, on your back, roll to the right . . . left leg somewhat balancing your weight . . . your right knee . . .
touches the floor . . . head goes close to the floor in the direction of the knee . . . the weight of the left leg enables you . . . to sit . . . in the position from which you started.

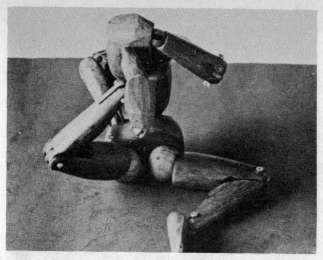

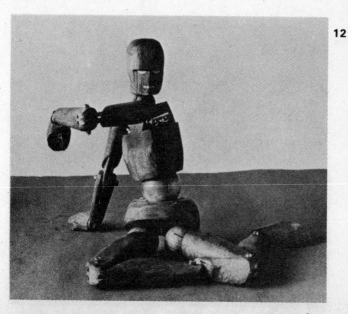

Lift that right foot in front of you . . . move it higher — higher — and at the top . . . curve it nearer to yourself . . . Lower your head; you will probably be able to bring that foot somewhere very near to the top of your head . . .

. . . move your hand and head, to the right . . . and from that position . . . move your head, with your eyes, back to the left . . . you look left.

13

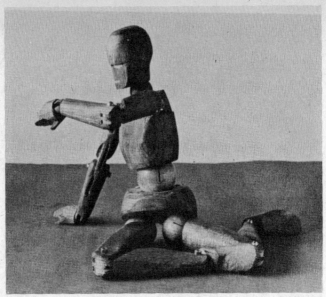

Sit on the floor. Lean on your right hand behind you . . . bend your left leg . . . to the left on to the floor near your buttock . . . the right foot near to yourself . . . somewhere near your left knee . . . Lift your left hand in front of . . . your eyes . . .

14

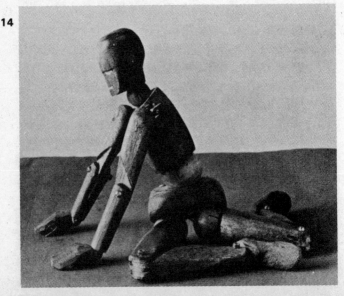

*. . . sit up again . . . turn both shoulders and head so that you can lean to the right on **both** hands . . .*

Lesson 5

Coordination of the Flexor Muscles and of the Extensors

Here you will learn to increase the contraction of the erector muscles of the back, and that prolonged contraction of the flexor muscles of the abdomen increases the tonus of the extensors of the back. You will be able to lengthen the muscles that twist the body. Lengthening the extensors of the nape by activating their antagonists in the front of the neck improves the balance of the head in the erect standing position. You will also learn improved differentiation of head and trunk movement.

The path of the stress in a twisting movement [Ill. 2]

Lie on your back; stretch out your legs, feet apart. Bend your knees and cross your legs, placing the right over the left.

Let both your knees drop down toward the right, so that both are now supported by the left foot only. The weight of the right leg will help both legs to sink to the right toward the floor. Now let your knees return to the neutral or middle position, then let them drop to the right again. Repeat twenty-five times. Your arms should be lying by the side of your body. Let your lungs fill with air as your knees return to the neutral position; breathe out as they sink down, so that each movement is completed in one breathing cycle.

Observe the movement of the pelvis as your legs sink down. The left side will rise a little from the floor and will be pulled in the direction of the left thigh; the spine will be pulled by the pelvis, and in its turn pull the chest with it until the left shoulder blade will tend to rise off the ground. Continue lowering the legs to the right until the left shoulder rises off the ground; then let the legs return to the middle. Try to observe the path by which the twisting movement is transmitted from the pelvis to the left shoulder, that is, through which vertebrae and ribs.

The movement of the spine is, of course, also felt in the movement of the head, the back of which is resting on the ground. As the knees sink down to right your chin will approach closer to the breastbone, and when the knees return to the middle, the head will lie flat as before.

Stretch out your legs, wait a moment, and try to feel on which side of your pelvis the change has been greater. One side lies flatter and its contact with the floor is more complete. Which side is it?

Movement of the knees [Ill. 3]

Draw up your knees, feet apart, and open your knees so that each is poised vertically above its foot. Better still, move the knees together and then pull them apart, and repeat until you can clearly feel when they are directly over the feet, that is, in the position in which no muscular effort is required to prevent them from either leaning against each other or falling apart.

Raise your arms in the direction of the ceiling above your eyes and place them together as if you were clapping your hands. Your shoulder, girdle, and arms will now form a triangle whose apex consists of your wrists, placed together. Raise your shoulder girdle from the floor as if someone were lifting your right shoulder. Both hands will now drop to the left, toward the floor. The previous triangle should remain unchanged, with no movement in the elbows; do not let your hands slip away from each other. Return to the middle. Breathe in, but without letting the pelvis move more than necessary.

Let the triangle formed by your arms drop toward the left as you breathe out. Repeat the whole movement twenty-five times.

See whether you must raise your head from the ground to carry out this movement and how far your arms will move to the left without your face also turning to the left.

Rest for a moment. Which shoulder is resting more firmly on the floor? Draw up your knees again. Place the right knee over the left, and let both sink down toward the right. See whether your knees will now drop lower than before or not.

Change your knees over, that is, cross the left over the right. Let both knees sink down to the left and bring them back to the middle. Repeat twenty-five times. Rest for a moment and observe which side is now closer to the floor and makes better contact with it.

Let the knees sink to the side again and observe how far and how easily they now sink down; you must do this in order to be able to observe improvement after the next stage has been completed, in which the upper part of the body will move.

Movement of the shoulder girdle to the right

Raise your hands to form a triangle as before. Let both arms drop to the right, and complete the twenty-five movements as you did before to the left.

Rest and observe the change in the contact of the shoulders with the floor.

Let your knees sink down to the left again and observe the improvement there has been as the result of the movement of the arms and shoulders to the right. The greater scope of the movement is due to the relaxation of the muscles between the ribs, which permits the spinal vertebrae to turn more freely.

Movement of the knees with simultaneous raising of head

Cross the right knee over the left. Let both knees sink to the right on their own, without any special effort. Link your hands behind your head with interlaced fingers and use your hands to help raise your head, letting the elbows approach close together in front while your head is raised. Then let your head return to rest on the floor, the elbows also returning to the floor. Let your lungs fill with air and raise your head again in the same way just as you begin to breathe out. Raise your head straight up in front, although your pelvis and legs are turned to the right.

Repeat twenty-five times, raising your head each time as you begin to breathe out. As you carry out this exercise observe the changes in floor contact of the ribs, spine, and pelvis. Rest a minute and observe which part of the trunk has sunk down to the floor most completely.

Interlace your fingers the other way

Cross your left knee over your right knee and let both knees sink to the left as far as feels comfortable. Interlace your fingers the opposite way from your usual position.

Now cross your fingers again without thinking—you probably obtain your habitual interlacing—then switch to the other and observe how this small change affects the positions of the shoulders and head. It may even seem to you that "everything is crooked."

Raise your head and repeat the previous movement, paying careful attention to all details. Rest after twenty-five such movements and observe the difference in the feeling of the contact your back makes with the floor.

Changes in the pelvic vertebrae

Lie on your back, draw up your knees, interlace your fingers behind your head, and raise it as you breathe out. Repeat twenty-five times. Rest for a few minutes lying on your back like this. Try to note in detail what changes have taken place in the hip vertebrae; it is possible that they may be lying flat on the floor for the first time in your life without any conscious effort. Perhaps they will only have sunk down a good way, for there is still some excess tension left in the muscles of the back that needs to be relaxed.

Rocking trunk with arms crossed [Ill. 4]

Lie on your back and draw up your knees so that your feet stand on the ground comfortably, well apart. Put your right hand under your left armpit on the left shoulder blade; pass your left hand under your right armpit to the right shoulder blade.

Now rock and roll your trunk to and fro from right to left and back, with your right hand lifting the left shoulder from the ground as you go to the right, and your left hand raising the right shoulder as you go to the left. Do not try to help the movement from the pelvis, but rock only the upper part of the body from one side to the other. Repeat twenty-five times, starting with a slow movement and increasing the speed until you are rolling freely in an easy rhythm.

Rest a moment. Change your arms over, so that the left hand is now under your right armpit and the right arm lies over your left arm. Do another twenty-five rolling movements in this position, starting slowly and then gathering speed.

Rocking movement with head still

Rest and try to remember whether your head has taken any part in these rocking movements from side to side. It almost certainly has. This time fix your eyes on some convenient spot on the ceiling. Hug your shoulders as before and repeat the rocking and rolling movement from side to side, keeping your pelvis still and your eyes fixed on the spot. This time your head will not take part in the rolling movement. This movement is unfamiliar, because you are not used to moving your shoulders without moving your head in the same direction.

Rest a minute and then repeat the rolling movement, but this time let your head move together with your shoulders. Now, while you continue the movement with your back, stop the head movement by again fixing your eyes on the ceiling. Observe the improvement in the rolling movement when you have learned to separate the movements of the head and shoulders.

Movement of head and shoulders in opposite directions

Rest. Then continue the rolling movements of the back as before, but this time turn your head and eyes in the opposite direction to that of the shoulders. Continue rolling the head and shoulders in opposite directions, making sure that the movement is well coordinated and smooth.

Reverse the position of your arms, putting the lower one on top, and do another twenty-five rolling movements with head and shoulders going in opposite directions. Then rest, and start again with head and shoulders moving together. Observe that the movement is now easier and more continuous although your rolling angle has grown.

Lie still. After a minute try to see whether there has been any further change in the spine. Is all of it now resting on the floor, including even the lumbar vertebrae?

Get up very slowly, walk a few steps, and observe the way in which you are now carrying your head as well as your breathing and the feeling in your shoulders. You will see that your whole body is more upright without any intentional effort. Consider these changes. Can you see how and why such major changes have taken place as the result of such simple movements for so short a time?

Lesson 6
Differentiation of Pelvic Movements by Means of an Imaginary Clock

In this lesson you will identify superfluous and unconscious efforts by the muscles of the pelvis and learn to refine control over the position of the pelvis and improve the alignment of the spine. You will increase your ability to coordinate and oppose head and trunk movements. This improves the twisting movements of the spine possible in the erect position. In primitive movements, eyes, head, and trunk turn right and left together. Awareness of this tendency makes it possible to turn each separately or in different combinations, making turning easier and increasing the maximum turning angle. You will also study the connection between the sensation caused by movement in the body and the location of the limbs in space.

Changing the lumbar curvature

Lie on your back, draw up your knees, and place your feet on the ground a comfortable distance apart, approximately in line with your hips. Place your hands on the ground on either side of your body, also a comfortable distance apart.

Raise your hips from the ground by an effort of the muscles of the back, so that the lumbar vertebrae form an arch on the floor. Try to make this arch larger, so that a mouse could run through

115

it. You will feel your feet gripping the floor. The muscles at the front of your hip joints will help by raising the upper part of your pelvis from the ground, resulting in increased pressure on the coccyx.

A clock dial on the pelvis

Imagine a clock dial painted on the back of your pelvis. The figure six is drawn on the coccyx and the twelve at the top of the pelvis where it joins the spine, a point that you can identify with your fingers (it is at the bottom of the fifth lumbar vertebrae). Keeping the imaginary dial in mind, we may say that in the movement just carried out the hips were raised and most of the pressure of the pelvis came to rest at the point marked six o'clock.

If we now complete the clock face, three o'clock will come in the area of the right hip joint, nine o'clock on the left hip joint. The other hours will be marked at their appropriate places in between.

Try once more to shift most of the pressure of the pelvis on the floor to the point marked six o'clock, the coccyx. Your back muscles will produce the curvature of the lumbar vertebrae, which will be increased by the contraction of the muscles of your pelvis and knees. This contraction pulls at your feet, which are still planted firmly on the floor.

Now shift most of the pressure to the point marked twelve o'clock. This means that the top of your pelvis and the lumbar vertebrae will now be resting on the ground. The coccyx will, of course, rise from the ground, and the pressure on your feet will increase.

Separate breathing from action

Return to six o'clock, then again to twelve o'clock, to and fro, and repeat twenty-five times. Gradually reduce the effort and make the change from one position to the other less jerky; also try to separate your breathing from the movement. Your breathing should continue quietly and easily without regard to the changes in the position of your body. The movements of the pelvis should be slow and continuous, with smooth changes from one position to the next.

Stretch out your legs and study the feeling in your pelvis. Try to observe accurately at which points contact with the floor is now different. Did you notice that as soon as your breathing was separated from the movement your head began to move in coordination with your pelvis as though it were "copying" the movement on a smaller scale?

A clock dial at the back of the head

Now let us imagine a small dial at the back of the head. The center of the dial will be at the point at which there is the greatest pressure when the head is resting on the ground. When the pelvis is in the position of maximum pressure at six o,clock, the head will be pulled down by the spine so that the chin comes to rest on the throat, and most of the pressure will now come at six o'clock on the head "dial." When the pelvic pressure comes at twelve o'clock, the head will be pushed back by the spine, the chin will be pushed away from the throat, and the point of maximum pressure will be shifted in the direction of the top of the head—at twelve o'clock on the head "dial."

Carry out the pelvic movements twenty-five times. Shift the weight of the pelvis from twelve o'clock to six o'clock and back again, but this time make sure that you are not preventing the head from repeating the movements of the pelvis.

Observe how this movement affects your breathing process and also how your trunk passes the movements of the pelvis on to your head, and the other way around. Rest a minute.

Draw your knees up again and lean the pelvis on the point marked three o'clock, on the right hip joint. You will now have more weight on your left foot than on your right, and the left hip joint will rise off the floor. The pressure on the right leg will be relaxed somewhat. Reverse the movement and lean on the point marked nine o'clock. Roll the pelvis from right to left and back again twenty-five times.

Observe how your head repeats this movement on a smaller scale as long as you do not tense your chest needlessly and do not interfere with the rhythm of your breathing. Rest a minute.

Around the clock in a continuous movement

Draw up your knees again. Rest your pelvis at twelve o'clock. Move the point of contact to one o'clock, and then return to twelve. Repeat five times. Now move your pelvis from twelve o'clock through one o'clock to two, and back again. Repeat five times. Now move its weight to three o'clock in the same way (through one and two).

Repeat each movement five times, then add a further hour and repeat again until you reach six o'clock, then repeat back to twelve. Each movement should mark a continuous arc, with no pause at the intermediate hours.

Observe how the awareness of the exact position reached by the pelvis gradually becomes more accurate and the weight moves round in a true arc, no longer in jerky straight movements from one point on the clock to the next.

Stop the movement, stretch out on the floor, and observe the difference between the right and left sides of the pelvis. While you are resting try to remember whether your head followed the movements of the pelvis on its own scale. We do many things without being aware of them.

Return to twelve o'clock. Shift the weight of the pelvis to eleven o'clock and back to twelve. Repeat five times. Move on to ten o'clock, through eleven, and back again. Continue as before, until you reach six o'clock. Rest a minute and observe what is happening in your body.

Lengthening the arcs

Shift most of the pressure of the pelvis to three o'clock, the right hip joint. Move the weight to four o'clock, return to three, move on to two. Then return from two to four through three and back. Repeat five times. Add one hour to each side of the movement.

The next movement will take you from one o'clock to five, and the one after from twelve to six. Repeat each movement five times.

Rest and observe the changes that have taken place in the contact of the pelvis with the floor as the result of this exercise.

Repeat this series of movements on the left side, with nine o'clock as the starting point.

Rest. Did you observe your head movements? Did you notice what your feet were doing, or any other part of your body?

The whole and its parts

Mark twenty circles on the floor with your pelvis, moving it clockwise. During this movement try to observe your body as a whole and at the same time its parts separately. Let your attention move systematically from one point of the body to the next, but without losing sight of your body as a whole. The sensation conveyed by your whole body will form only a background and will be less clear, of course. It is somewhat like what we do when we read: We see the whole page at a glance, but this impression is not sufficiently clear for comprehension; we can grasp the meaning only of those letters and words that we have seen clearly.

Observe the movements of your head without stopping the clockwise movements of both pelvis and head. Concentrate alternately on your head as leading the movement, then on the pelvis as leading it. Observe how the quality of the movement improves steadily, becoming more continuous, smoother, more accurate, and faster.

Rest. Make twenty counterclockwise movements of the pelvis and head.

Consider objective versus subjective judgment

Up to now we have imagined the dial as drawn on the body itself at points identified by pressure on the floor. Now imagine the six and twelve of the dial drawn on the floor and mentally measure the distance between them. Mentally measure the same distance on your body, and note how different the sense of distance is in the two cases. Which is more concrete? Which is correct? In the first case (the floor), your judgment is more objective; in the second, on your body, it is more subjective.

As you proceed with this lesson you will discover that your judgment is different in the two cases, but that the subjective evaluation converges on the objective evaluation asymptotically. In other words, the subjective sensation has a wider field of operation than objective evaluation, which limits our capacity for knowledge to the simple material reality around us. Concrete reality imposes necessary limits, but it is the lowest common denominator that serves all of us. The true capacity of any nervous system can be estimated only by its individual characteristics— that is, man's own personality. By this test the differences between individuals are enormous. When these concepts are more widely accepted the general level will rise, and therefore the span of differences between individuals will grow even more.

Inner and outer contact

Carry out the circular clockwise movement with your pelvis again. This time imagine that the figures of the dial on your body protrude a little and as the pressure point passes them they leave an imprint on the floor, like a rubber stamp. Follow the contact of each figure on your pelvis and its imprint on the floor below. This is what I have named the establishing of inner and outer contact alternately, until these are combined in a single essential operation.

Rest. As usual, observe the changes that have taken place in the position of the whole body with respect to the floor.

Repeat the exercise with the pelvis moving counterclockwise. Rest and remember how your body lay on the floor at the beginning of the lesson and mentally identify the changes. The improvement will seem to you to have reached its peak now, and your pelvis should be lying flat and close to the ground both lengthwise and crosswise. But this is not the case, for in fact there is no limit to improvement of action.

More pelvic rotations

Draw up your right knee, the left leg remaining stretched out and at an angle. Make twenty clockwise pelvic movements. Note which "hours" are pressing more strongly on the floor than before, which less strongly.

Make twenty counterclockwise pelvic movements with your left knee bent and check which hours have become more clearly marked. Those less clearly marked now will be symmetrical with those that are less clear when the right knee is bent.

Stretch out your legs and observe whether there has been any further change in the contact of your pelvis with the floor. You will discover once more that it is only after changes have taken place that we can observe clearly what the position was before.

Lie on the floor with your feet apart and make clockwise circular movements with your pelvis. Check in which positions it now presses down more strongly and in which less strongly. Reverse the direction of the movement and note the difference.

Cross your right leg over your left knee. Make twenty clockwise movements and then twenty counterclockwise ones. Rest and check the results. Cross the left leg over the right knee, and repeat as before.

Very, very slowly, after resting at least a full minute, roll on one side and stand up. Observe the changes in the angle of the pelvis with respect to the spine, the quality of your breathing, and the movement of your arms and legs. What can you feel in your eyes and your facial muscles?

What happens in the next stage?

At a later stage the body positions used here will serve as new patterns of movement, for we shall learn to move the head and pelvis in opposite directions. When the head moves clockwise, the pelvis will move counterclockwise. This will produce changes that improve the body image, the relationship of its parts to each other, and the continuity of the movement. This means that the degree of control is increased still further.

When awareness is further developed we shall add one more element, namely, the movement of the eyes. They can move together with the pelvis in the opposite direction to the head itself, or else together with the head, in the direction opposite to that of the pelvic movement. As awareness matures, the limits of understanding expand.

Other positions may be tried for the pelvis moving around a dial, such as propping oneself up with the forearms, with the knees open and flexed so that the soles of the feet touch each other; or sitting and propping oneself up with the hands on the floor behind the body. In each of these positions numerous variations can be used.

Lesson 7

The Carriage of the Head Affects the State of the Musculature

In this lesson you will study the dependence of all the muscles in your body on the work of the muscles of the head and neck. (The freer and easier the movements of your head become, and the farther it can turn, the easier it will become to turn your whole body as far as it is anatomically possible.) You will discover the immediate effects of imagined movements and learn to distinguish between the projected image of an action and its actual execution, and thus acquire improved gradation of muscular effort. You will find that awareness of the differentiation between the projected image of a movement and its execution is a means to finer muscular action.

Rotation of legs to the right [Ill. 5]

Lie on your stomach. Place the palms of your hands on the floor, one on top of the other, so that you can rest your forehead on them. Place your feet apart about the width of your hips. Raise your feet from the floor by bending your knees, and lean one foot against the other. Your knees will form approximately a right angle with the thighs and be wide apart; the soles of your feet will face the ceiling.

Rotate your legs to your right; i.e. let them sink toward the floor, but without allowing the left knee to rise from the floor. In order to make this possible, the left foot must slide along the right ankle and leg, while the right foot approaches the ground. When your legs return to the starting position, the left foot will slide back along the right leg past the ankle to come to rest next to the right foot. Repeat these movements twenty-five times and observe meanwhile through which parts of the bone structure of your body the turning movement is passed on from the legs to the vertebrae of the neck.

Observe which of your elbows is pulled somewhat down farther in the direction of the legs during the movement to the right and how this elbow returns to its original position as the feet return to the middle. The movement of the elbow is quite small, of course, but large enough to be noticeable.

Face left during leg movement to the right

Place your left palm on the back of your right hand; turn your head to the left and let your right ear and right cheek rest on your hands. Again, bend your knees and let your legs sink to the right and then let them return to the middle. Observe your ribs in front and note the growing pressure on one side of the breastbone as your legs come down to the right. Adjust your position by relaxing your chest so as to reduce the pressure on the ribs, and let the pressure spread over a larger area until you have reduced it to a minimum. With every leg movement, follow its effects from vertebra to vertebra in the direction of the head, and check whether the turning movement is regular or whether whole groups of vertebrae move together in some sections instead of moving one after the other. Note whether the leg movement became larger when you turned your head to the left.

Check by lying on your back

After twenty-five movements rest on your back and check the whole of your trunk to see whether there are any changes in its contact with the floor. Turn your head from right to left on the floor several times and observe whether there is any difference between its movements to the two sides, that is, whether your face turns to the right more easily, smoothly, and in a wider arc than to the left, or less well.

Face and legs to the right

Lie on your stomach again. Place the palm of your left hand on your right hand. Turn your head to the right so that your left cheek and ear rest on the top hand. Continue to rotate your lower legs down to the right, making sure that you do not change the distance between the knees during this movement. Let the left foot slide along the right leg as before.

Observe whether the degree of twist in the spine is larger or smaller now, whether it is easier or more difficult to move the legs sideways, and whether turning the head to the right tends to obstruct or aid the leg movement.

Twisting of spine and breathing

Imagine a finger traveling along your spine, from the coccyx to the base of the skull, stopping to mark each separate vertebra on the way. It is easier in this way to check whether there is any movement at all in the vertebrae, to see where the twist is gradual and where more strongly marked. Note the moment in the movement at which your lungs fill with air: Is it while your legs return to the neutral position in the middle or during the active phase, when you are rotating your legs? For an easier and more extensive twist while lying on the floor, your chest should be empty of air and your rib muscles relaxed. Rest for a minute on your back.

Head immobile and knees joined together

Lie on your stomach. Turn your head to the left and rest your right ear and cheek on the floor. Interlace the fingers of your hands and place them over your left ear, resting your elbows on the floor on either side of your head. This position is intended to let the frame formed by your arms exert gentle but continuous pressure on the left side of your face, thereby gradually increasing the angle at which your head is turned sideways. The weight of your arms itself only helps you to feel the change that has actually been brought about by the work of the trunk in easing the movement of the vertebrae. Put your knees together and bend them at approximately a right angle. The soles of your feet are now turned to the ceiling.

Incline both legs to the right, but this time make sure that they remain together, as though they were tied together at the knees and ankles. You will find that you are now able to incline your legs to the right only if your left knee and thigh leave the floor. Return to the middle, then incline the legs again. Repeat twenty-five times.

Soften your body

Time the leg movement so that it begins as you exhale. Note the gradual twist that has taken place along the whole length of your spine, with particular attention for the upper chest vertebrae and the lower vertebrae of the nape. The twisting of the pelvis will cause stretching in the spine. Note the movement felt in the left elbow, and at every movement try to lengthen your body and to make the action of the legs smoother and rounder. Pay special attention to this when you change the direction of the leg movement.

Changes in the movement of the head

When you have finished these movements let your head return very gradually to the central position. The changes that have taken place in the neck vertebrae and in the muscles of the nape may be so great that the first normal movement carried out at this stage, without taking the changes into account, is liable to be most unpleasant. But after the first careful, slow movement there is no need for further special care; on the contrary, the movement of the head in the direction in which this exercise was carried out has improved quite unmistakably.

Lie on your back, let your head rest on the floor and turn it to the right and the left. Observe whether the movement really has improved and has become more continuous and smoother in the direction in which it turned during the last exercise, and is also turning through a wider angle on that side than the other.

Get rid of the old when you have new

The discomfort, or even pain, experienced during normal behavior after a large number of successive movements in one particular position is interesting. We are unable to use our bodies in any but accustomed patterns of muscular action. When extensive change is introduced to most of the muscles, or at least to those essential to the movement carried out—as with twenty-five repetitions of a movement—we nevertheless instruct our muscles to fall into their usual pattern.

Only the experience of change and close attention will convince us to think and direct ourselves differently. Only when this experience of change causes us to discredit and inhibit the accustomed pattern, which now appears invalid to us, will we be able to accept the new pattern as habit or second nature. Theoretically, all that is needed is an effort of the mind, but in practice this is insufficient. Our nervous system is so constructed that habits are preserved and seek to perpetuate themselves. It is easier to stop a habit by means of a sudden traumatic shock than to change it gradually. This is a functional difficulty, and that is why it is important to pay close attention to every improvement and to assimilate it after every series of movements. We thus get a double effect on our sensing capacity: the inhibition of the previous, automatic pattern of movement, which now feels wrong, heavy, and less comfortable, and the encouragement of the new pattern, which will appear more acceptable, more flowing, and more satisfactory. The insight thus obtained is not an intellectual one—proven, understood, and convincing—but a matter of deeper sensing, the fruit of individual experience. It is important to know and understand the connection between the change and its causes in order to encourage one to repeat the experience with sufficient accuracy under similar conditions to reinforce its effect and impress the improvement deeply on our senses.

Stronger twisting movement

Lie on your stomach again and turn your head to the right, resting your left cheek on the floor. Interlace your fingers the unfamiliar way; rest your hands so folded on your right ear, join your knees together, and bend them at a right angle as before. Now incline your legs down toward the floor on the right side. Your right thigh and knee will turn on their outer side each time that the legs approach the floor. There is a discernible twisting effect on the neck vertebrae, and of course your legs need not come down as far as the floor at first, even if it is possible but uncomfortable. Continue to improve the movement gradually, repeating it twenty-five times. Meanwhile, observe your entire body carefully.

Differences in sensing and movement on the two sides of the body.

Rest. Observe the difference felt in lying on your back now compared to the beginning of the lesson. Get up, walk about a little, and observe the different feeling in the movements of the head, the erect position of the trunk, the control of the legs, breathing, and the position of the pelvis. See whether you can sense any difference in the feeling between the right eye and the left. Look in a mirror to see whether there is any objective difference in your face to show on which side the leg exercise was carried out.

Lie on your stomach again. Rest your forehead on your hands and incline your legs to the right in the simplest manner possible. They will now either reach the floor or at least be nearer to it, and

their movement will be much easier and smoother than before you
began this lesson.

Lie on your back and check the contact made with the floor by
the two sides of your body from your heels to the top of your head.

Mental recall

Lie down on your stomach again. Rehearse in your mind all the
different movements that you have practiced in this lesson. This
is not very difficult, because we progressed from the simple to the
more elaborate, twisting the spine from its two ends, from the
nape and from the pelvis.

When you can remember it all quite clearly, work through all
the symmetrical positions with your legs moving to the left, but
in your mind only. That is, imagine the sensation of these movements in your muscles and bones, going just so far as to tense the
muscles slightly, but not making any visible movement. This
method becomes effective much more quickly. It is sufficient to
think each movement only five times, but you will have to count
the movements in order not to daydream. It is difficult to concentrate without any action; it is more difficult to think than to act,
and indeed, most people would rather do than think what they are
doing.

Rest after every five imaginary movements and check the result.

Awareness of self-image

Slowly you will become aware of a strange sensation, unfamiliar
to most people: a clearer picture of your self-image. Here the new
image concerns mainly the muscles and skeletal structure. It is
much more complete and accurate than that to which you were
accustomed and you wonder why you did not learn of this condition sooner.

Lie on your stomach and observe on which side the movement
is better: on the side on which you did so much practicing, or on
that on which you did so little thinking.

In this lesson you will learn to use a group of muscles for a specific movement in various positions of the body. You will make the joints employed in this movement more flexible and reach the anatomically possible limits within the first hour. You will learn the effect of movements of the head on muscular tension, the effect of imagined movement on real movement, and to inhibit verbalization in imagined movement—all of which leads to completion of the body image. You will also be able to transfer improvement actively obtained by one side of the body to the other inactive side, which did not take part in the movement, by means of visualization or thought only.

Raise the foot in the direction of your head [Ill. 6]

Sit on the floor with your knees opened out and your feet resting on their outside edges in front of you. Place your right hand under your right heel so that your heel rests in the palm of your hand. To do this, raise the heel a little from the floor, and push the hand like a wedge between the floor and the heel. Keep the thumb together with the fingers, which grip the heel. Now take hold of the four small toes of your right foot with your left hand, with the left thumb passing between the big toe and that next to it. Close your left hand. The small toes will be held in the grip of the left hand. [Ill. 7]

Raise your right foot with the aid of both hands and at the same time push it away from your body. Then pull it toward your head in a well-rounded movement; then lower it to its original position. Repeat, raising your leg as you breathe out. Drop your head forward as far as is comfortable to allow your leg, which will slowly be raised well above the head, to complete its movement toward the body smoothly before it returns to the floor.

Continue raising the leg, but without strain, without trying too hard, and without forcing the movement. Simply repeat the movement, making it smoother and easier each time, more continuous and more comfortable to carry out. Observe your chest, shoulders, and shoulder blades, and stop "trying." "Trying" prevents the movement from becoming easier and wider. In a skeleton without muscles one would not experience the least difficulty in raising the foot high and letting it come to rest on the top of its head. The muscles form the chief obstacle to this movement, because some of them continue to be tensed and shorter than their true anatomical length, even in a state of complete rest.

Repeat this movement about twenty times, then lie on the floor to rest.

Action without awareness

When you rest after a movement carried out without much effort, it is not in order to regain strength, but to study the changes that have taken place during the action. It takes a minute or two, or even longer, before it is possible to observe these changes. The result is that people who are accustomed to switch from one action to another without sufficient pause in between fail to observe the aftereffects of a series of repeated movements. Many teachers do not give their students the time needed to detect the aftereffects of various actions, even such abstract ones as thinking.

Using muscles without observation, discrimination, and understanding is merely machinelike movement, of no value except for its
produce; it could also be obtained from a donkey or even a real machine. Such work does not call for the highly developed human nervous system. The reception of abstract mental impressions remains a
mere mechanical process unless time is allowed to let the individual
become aware of the fact that he is paying attention and that this
attention is sufficient for understanding. Without this, the impressions will remain a mere recording. The result will at best be a mechanical repetition of the mental process, but without its becoming
an integrated part of the personality.

Raising of foot while lying on back [Ill. 8]

Lie on your back and draw up your feet with knees open as
before. Raise your right foot, and with both arms between your
knees, grip it as before: the right hand under the heel, with all
fingers and also the thumb under the heel, and the left hand
holding the four smaller toes. Use your hands to lift your foot in
a smooth movement away from your body, in the direction of the
ceiling. Now let the path of the foot curve toward the head,
meanwhile raising the head as though to meet the foot. Lower the
foot to a comfortable position, but without letting go of it. Repeat
twenty-five times, but without forcing the movement.

Select a path through the air for your foot that will make for
a light and gentle movement. You will succeed if you do it without
any determination to do it better. Observe the changes in the
foot's path and the various strains in the chest and arms. Stop and
rest on your back.

Draw your knees up again and once more grip your right foot
with both hands. Let your left foot rest easily on the floor. Use
your hands to move your right foot away from your body, then turn
the pelvis to the right until the right thigh touches the floor. The
head and body will also turn to the right. As you breathe out, bend

to bring your head forward in the direction of the right knee in a large arc close to the floor, in order to try to bring the body into a sitting position.

Try once more. Let your left leg help by rising off the floor, stretching, and then moving back and a little to the left, the knee folding up as you try to sit. It is not necessary or important that you should succeed at the first or second attempt. In any case lie down again on your back and try to turn over to the right lightly, without special effort.

Head movement in an arc close to the floor

Continue with the head movement close to the floor, and use your hands to pull your right foot gently in such a way that it helps your head to mark its arc closer to the floor, and toward an imaginary point on the floor, in front of the knee and a little to the right of it. Use your left leg to help you as before. Remember to keep your chest relaxed, to try less hard, and to observe those parts of the body in which there is muscular effort that does not become transformed into movement.

Repeat several times. Each time observe the parts of your body that are missing in the body image of the movement and try to complete the image.

Try this twenty-five times, but do not expect that there will be results from each movement. Rest for about two minutes.

Rocking movement of trunk from side to side

Sit, and spread your bent knees apart. Stretch your arms out between your legs, and grip your right foot as before. Raise your foot forward and upward over your head, and see whether there has been any improvement.

Without letting go of your right foot, place your left leg behind you on the left, with the inside of the foot and knee on the ground. At the same time place your right foot on the floor in front of you.

Your head will sink down forward together with the trunk. Bring it closer to the floor in front of you in whatever direction is most comfortable, in front of the right knee or lower leg. Rock the trunk from right to left in the smallest movements that seem comfortable to you.

Rolling from sitting to lying positions and back, on the right side [Ills. 9 and 10]

After a few small movements increase the rocking motion until, with lowering your head, you succeed in rolling to the right on the floor until you are lying on your back. Your left foot will, of course, also rise from the ground. If the movement was fairly comfortable and smooth you will pass through the lying position on your back and find yourself lying almost on your left side.

Push away from the floor with your left foot and begin the movement back to the right. Fold up your body and roll with your head leading and kept close to the ground until it reaches the right knee. If you remember to fold your left leg behind you, to the left of the body, you will be certain to reach the sitting position again.

Be careful not to straighten up as you reach the sitting position, but to keep your head and trunk as close to the floor as possible. In this position move the body a little to the left by means of a movement of the trunk and head to give you a start, and roll again to the right until you are lying on your back. Repeat the rolling movement twenty-five times, then rest.

Repeat, but in imagination only

If you did not succeed in rolling from the lying to the sitting position and back again, try to carry out the movement in your imagination both while lying on your back and while sitting, five times in each position, attending to as many parts of your body as you can. Observe the imagined movement and make sure it is continuous. Make sure your breathing retains its quiet rhythm and then try the real movement again.

Raising foot while sitting, in fact and in imagination [Ill. 11]

Sit as at the beginning of the lesson. Hold your foot as before and try to raise it over your head, using both hands, and to rest it on the top of your head. No effort is needed in a well-organized body in order to place the hollow at the inside edge of the foot on the top of the head. If you have difficulty in carrying this out, sit with closed eyes and visualize the movement in detail, and as one continuous movement. Note how difficult it is to imagine how a movement will feel if you cannot carry it out.

Verbalization can take the place of sensation and control

Of course there is no difficulty at all in thinking the movement in words. One of the great disadvantages of the spoken language is the fact that it permits us to become estranged from our real selves to such an extent that we often have the mistaken belief that we have imagined something, or thought of something, where in reality we have only recalled the appropriate word. It is a simple matter to confirm for ourselves that when we really imagine an action we come up against the same obstacles as in performing the action itself. It is difficult to carry out a particular action because the orders of the nervous system to the muscles do not fit the action. The body will not fold up closely enough because the conscious instruction for the folding up cannot be carried out, and because the antagonist muscles—those that serve to straighten the back, in this case—continue to work too hard as a matter of habit resulting from poor posture. It is enough for their obstructive activity to become consciously aware, for a new flexibility to appear suddenly, a flexibility like that of an infant, and the folding movement to become continuous, comfortable, miraculous.

The moment this happens the individual feels as though a window had opened into a dark room and he is filled with a new feeling of ability and life. He has discovered mastery of himself, and realizes that responsibility for his uncontrolled movements rests largely with himself.

Complete your body image

Close your eyes and think through all the positions listed in this lesson. Observe the feeling in your limbs during each "movement," and repeat it two or three times in each position, with ample pauses between one movement and the next. Then try to lift your foot again and observe whether it now obeys your wish to lift it over your head more easily, and whether you can now rest it on the top of your head.

There is no limit to improvement

It may be that the obstructions to movement have become so great that it is not possible to reach the change described above in the course of a single lesson without a teacher. With personal instruction in groups of forty to fifty men and woman of all ages (often over sixty), it is a fact that 90 percent of those present get at least as far as touching their big toes to their foreheads, and the majority get as far as it is at all possible to get by now: placing the foot on the top of the head. All show notable improvement, and that is what matters. If it is possible for a person to reach a condition in which he registers improvement every time he does something, there is no limit to his possible achievement.

Repeat all movements to the left in imagination

Get up and walk about and observe the difference in sensation between the side observed during the exercises and the other side. Study the face, eyes, movement, and turns from side to side.

Lie on your back and simply draw up your knees. Close your eyes and observe the difference in the contact with the floor between the right and left sides. Imagine all the stages of movement in this lesson on the left side instead of the right, but imagine the sensation, not words. Repeat each imaginary movement three times, with good pauses between each movement and the next.

Improvement is greater through visualization than through action

Now sit up and grip your left foot with both hands in a symmetrical position to that taken up before; lift the foot over your head and try to place it on top of your head. You will certainly discover that the side on which you only imagined the exercises will obey you better and work better than the side on which you actually carried them out.

The side that actually worked also carried out many wrong or bad movements, which is usual when a new movement is tried, and therefore the achievement on the second side is greater and better.

Observing the self is better than mechanical repetition

Study the importance of this conclusion. You worked a full hour on one side, and spent only a few minutes on the second—and that only in the imagination—but nevertheless the improvement on the second side was greater. Yet all methods of gymnastics are based on the repetition of action. And not only gymnastics—everything we learn is based largely on the principle of repetition and committing to memory. This may make it easier to understand why one man may practice daily on a musical instrument and fail to make any progress, while another shows daily improvement. Perhaps the nature of the talent that is the accepted explanation for this divergence of achievement derives from the fact that the second student observes what he is doing while he plays while the first one only repeats and memorizes and relies on the assumption that sufficient repetition of a bad performance will somehow bring about musical perfection.

We have earlier referred to the concept of internal and external contact, which includes the transfer of conscious observation from the sensation inside the body to its changes in space outside it. Consider what a painter does when he studies a landscape and tries to draw it on his canvas. Can he do it without paying attention to the feeling in his hand as it directs the paintbrush? Can he do it without an awareness of what his eyes are seeing?

We have all experienced an occasion while reading when we had to go back and reread a passage because we read it the first time without paying attention. Although we probably read every word the first time, and even formed the words voicelessly, we did not understand or retain anything. What are we actually noticing during the second reading? Does it really make that much difference that we should observe the workings of our mind while reading?

Lesson 9

Spatial Relationships as a Means to Coordinated Action

You will now learn that conscious attention to the spatial relationships between moving limbs makes movement coordinated and flowing, and attentive systematic scanning of a part of the body can relax superfluous muscular tension there. Mechanical action does not teach us anything and will not improve ability. Common movements carried out in a different way most often indicate poor coordination, not superior individual ability. In fact, as movement improves it will approximate more closely the usual movement carried out by most people.

A clock opposite your face

Sit on the floor, legs crossed or not, with your knees apart in a comfortable position. Put your hands behind you so that you can lean on them. Imagine the numbered dial of a clock opposite your face and move your nose in a circular path as though you wanted to push the hands of the clock around the dial clockwise. The circle your nose will make must be small, for in a larger circle your nose would lose contact with the clock hands at the extreme right and extreme left of the dial. Continue this simple movement very slowly, many times, and make sure it does not interfere with your breathing.

Path of the ear lobe

Imagine that the lobe of your left ear is connected by a thin rubber band to the edge of your left shoulder. Decide in which part of the movement the rubber band stretches and becomes longer and when it becomes shorter, and by how much. The movement of the nose is circular and carried out at an even speed. Is the movement of the ear lobe also circular? Try to guess where your ear lobe will be when your nose is at twelve o'clock, three, six, nine, and again at twelve. Repeat this many times, always more and more quietly. Try to keep track of the ear lobe by feeling only: Simply pay attention until you can feel clearly where the ear lobe is in relationship to the edge of the shoulder.

We may act without knowing what we are doing

The preceding action is not simple. You will not succeed immediately, and there is no reason why you should. Such a solution would be a purely intellectual one, built on geometrical formulas you have learned; this will add nothing to your awareness. But is it not surprising that something so unclear can be going on in one part of your head while what you are doing with another part is perfectly clear? Apparently we may do things without knowing that we are doing them. It is a fact that we do not sense all the movements made by the head while we are thinking about one particular aspect of the movement.

Shift the focus from ear lobe to nose and back

Continue the movement of your nose and, without interrupting it, shift the focus of your attention to the ear lobe. Draw imaginary circles with your ear lobe in such a way that the nose can continue its regular movements. In what direction is the ear moving? Observe what is happening now to the rubber band that links your ear lobe to the shoulder; the movement is not the same as before. Has your nose changed its path, is it still drawing circles? Return your attention to your nose and let it move in a circle. Check the path of your ear lobe again. We might have assumed that as the nose and ear are both parts of the same head, if one part draws a circle the other (and the rest of the head with it) would also draw circles. But it seems the matter is not this simple.

Look with your left eye

Reverse the direction of the circles made by your nose so that it will push the hands around counterclockwise. Close both eyes and focus your attention on the left one. Where do you really look with this eye? Try to look with your closed left eye toward the bridge of your nose, between the two eyes, and then outward, toward the left corner of your left eye, while you continue to make circular movements with your nose. Most people give up after they have tried this a few times and have not succeeded in finding a clear answer. Perhaps we can find the answer only after we have become accustomed to the movement.

Try to move your left eye in a circle and find out how this affects the circles with your nose. Rest.

Color the left half of your head with an imaginary paintbrush

Sit comfortably on the floor with your legs crossed. Make clockwise circles with your nose and at the same time try to color the left half of your head with an imaginary paintbrush about two fingers wide. Imagine your left hand holding the brush and moving it first from the large shoulder vertebra to the left side of the nape, making a band two fingers wide along the neck and back of the head to the left of the line dividing it in half. Continue from the top of the head to the face, the forehead, the left eye, cheek, upper lip, lower lip, chin, round underneath the lower jaw on the left side of the neck to the collarbone; go back again, in the same way, to the back of the neck. Continue to go over the whole left half of the face and head, to the left shoulder, in adjacent bands of color.

Move nose to the right as you color the left half of the head

Rest a moment and then reverse the direction of movement of the nose. Color the left half of the head again, but with strokes at right angles to the earlier strokes—that is, with strokes going from the right to the left and back, so that the whole left half of the head and face have been covered a second time. See whether the painting movements interfere with the movements of the nose, and if so, at which points? When the brush is changing its direction? Is the passage of the brush sensed equally at all points, or are there places that remain unclear as the brush passes over them? Or where breathing is interfered with? In which places were there muscular tension and breaks in the movement? In the eye? Neck? Shoulders? Diaphragm? Rest.

Shifting attention from part to part

Continue the counterclockwise nose movements. During the movement decide that you want to draw circles with your chin. After a few minutes decide that you are really moving the corner of your left jaw, just under the ear. Then shift your attention to the left temple, and then to a point between the ear and the neck vertebrae at the base of the head.

After every five or ten head movements imagine that you transfer the center of movement to another section of the head, one after the other, but between each return to the nose. Continue until it becomes possible to include all parts of the left side of the head and face in a single mental effort with equal clarity. Rest.

Kneel with the right foot on the ground

Kneel on your left knee with your right foot standing on the ground. Stretch your right arm out in front of you and your left arm behind you, both at shoulder level. Close your eyes and imagine a thin rubber band connecting your left ear to your left hand (which is stretched out backward) and a second rubber band that connects it to your right hand (which is stretched out in front). Make twenty-five circular movements with your nose in one direction and another twenty-five in the opposite direction, and try to follow the shortening and lengthening of the two rubber bands in space.

Left foot on the ground

After a short rest return to a kneeling position with the left foot on the ground; stretch out your left hand in front and your right hand behind, at shoulder height. Repeat the nose movements and continue to observe the movements of the rubber bands.

Get up and walk about. Can you feel a difference when holding your head on the right or left side? Is the feeling of space different on the two sides? Is there a different feeling in the toes of the right and left foot?

Calisthenics for their own sake teach nothing

All the movements that we have made were symmetrical both in terms of space and with respect to the muscles, so what has caused these differences between right and left? We have made exactly the same movements on the left side, exactly the same number of times, but there is hardly any change on this side. It may be difficult to remember what the right side felt like before, and perhaps we cannot rely on our memory, but there is no doubt that the left side feels different from the right one. Does this not mean that movement by itself is worth very little? Most of the change has taken place on the side to which conscious attention was given. Must we assume that mechanical repetition has no value except to the extent that it stimulates circulation and uses the muscles? Is this why people who do gymnastics all their lives are not much more successful in any constructive activity than those who do not? There are people, on the other hand, who continue to observe the feeling in their body as they did during their period of growth, and they thus continue to learn and change and develop throughout their lives.

Individual movement becomes generalized

The differences in simple head movement as performed by different people derive from the fact that one person may attend to his ear as he turns his head and considers that the required movement, another may attend to the configuration of his ear and shoulder, and a third to the folding of the skin of his neck. The number of possible combinations here is so great that any movement will appear to be entirely personal and specific.

In a large group of students a great variety of head movements can be seen when the circular movement of the nose is first attempted, some so unusual as to seem incredible. By the end of the lesson a more general, common movement can be observed. The nose is really drawing circles accurately, both in subjective feeling and in reality. When the self-image is clearly present in the awareness of the individual during the movement, and when both objective and subjective impressions or representations are scanned as easily as looking at an object with our eyes, then the action becomes easy, accurate, and pleasant. It has also come closer to the movements carried out by any person with a developed awareness. Individuality should express itself in positive values, not in peculiarities.

Lesson 10

The Movement of the Eyes Organizes the Movement of the Body

Now you will learn how eye movements coordinate the body movements, and how they are linked to the movement of the neck muscles. Testing these connections of eye and neck muscles separately increases control of body movements and makes them easier. The movement of the eyes in an opposite direction to that of the head—and movement of the head in an opposite direction to that of the body—add a dimension of movement of which many are not aware. These exercises broaden the spectrum of activity and help to eliminate faulty habits of movement. You will also be able to distinguish between the muscles that control the movement of the eyeballs and the muscles that control vision more specifically.

Movement to the right and the left while standing

Stand with your feet slightly apart and swing your body to the right and to the left with your hands hanging limp at your sides. As you swing to the right, your right hand moves to the right behind the back and the left hand moves to the right in front of the body, as though it were trying to overtake the right elbow. As you swing to the left, your left hand moves to the left behind the

body, and the right hand moves to the left and overtakes it in
front.

Continue the swinging movements of the body and close your
eyes. Make sure that the movements of the head are smooth. At
each change of direction see what starts to turn back first: the eyes,
the head, or the pelvis. Make many such swinging movements,
from right to left and back again, until the answer is clear to you
and you can observe all your members during the movement
without stopping at the beginning or the end of the swing.

Open your eyes and go on swinging as before. Note whether
your eyes continue to look toward your nose, as when they were
closed, or whether they do something else—and if so, what are
they doing? Do they anticipate the movements of the head? Do
they skip parts of the horizon of vision?

Coordination of the eyes and fluidity of movement [Ill. 12]

Close your eyes again and try to sense when the swinging
movements are smoother and more fluent, when the eyes are
open or shut. Try to achieve with open eyes the degree of
smoothness attained with shut eyes. One would expect the
movement to be better in every respect when the eyes are
open, but it appears in practice that this often leads to inter-
ruptions in the fluidity of movement and its extent, owing to
the fact that the eye movements of many people are not properly coordinated with their muscular activity. Note carefully
the sensation of the movements of the legs and the pelvis and
all the minor flaws in the swinging movement in order to become aware of the changes that will be produced in the control of all the movements of the body.

Turning the body to the right while sitting [Ill. 13]

Sit on the floor. Bend the left leg backward to the left; the inside
of the left leg will rest on the floor with the left foot on its side.
Lean the palm of the right hand on the floor. Draw your right foot

toward your body so that the right calf lies parallel to the front of the body and the sole touches the thigh near the left knee. Stretch your left hand forward, opposite the eyes, and turn your trunk to the right with the left hand leading. With your eyes follow the thumb of the hand in its movement to the right.

Return to the middle and then turn to the right again, within the limit of comfort. Bend the left elbow so that the palm will be able to move farther to the right. Make sure that the eyes remain at rest, that is, fixed on the palm of the hand as the head and shoulders move to the right. Continue moving slowly, without trying to go farther to the right than is comfortable. Make sure that your eyes do not move farther right than your head carries them. Try not to shorten the spine, that is, not stiffen the chest and the ribs, allowing the head to ride high without making any effort to sit more upright intentionally. Be careful to let the eyes follow the palm of the left hand as it moves. Many people unconsciously go on looking farther to the right even after the hand has stopped moving, sometimes even after this has been pointed out to them.

Lie down to rest, and check the contact of your back with the floor.

Turning the trunk to the left while sitting

Sit and move both feet to the right in a position symmetrical to the last one. Stretch your right arm in front of your eyes and turn your entire trunk to the left as the eyes follow the thumb of your hand. Bend the right elbow as the hand moves to the left, so that it can reach farther to the left. Return to the starting position and make twenty-five turns to the left, making each movement easier than those before it. Pay attention to the movement itself and to its quality, not to moving farther to the left. Note the pelvis, the spine, the nape, any excessive stiffness in the ribs, and whatever else may interfere with the ease with which the movement is performed. Lie on your back and rest.

Eye movement widens the turning angle

Sit and bend your left leg backward to the left. Draw the right leg along the floor near the body. Turn the trunk to the right and lean on the right hand on the floor. The hand thus lies farther to the right than before because the trunk has already turned to the right. Lift the left arm to the front, before the eyes, and, with a movement of the trunk, carry it to the right. Bend the left elbow in such a way as to bring the left hand as far to the right as is comfortable and remain there.

In this twisted position of the trunk move the eyes to the right of the left hand, and then bring them back to rest on the hand. Move your eyes in this way—to the right of the hand and back again—some twenty times. Use the head movement to guide the direction of your gaze. Make sure that the eye movements remain horizontal, since they tend to drop downward at the extreme right of the path.

Don't shorten your body

In order to facilitate this movement, be careful to avoid shortening the neck. The spine must move lightly, as though someone were helping you by easing your head upward from above by gently pulling the hair at the top of your head. You can also ease the movement by lifting the left ischium (buttock bone) off the floor. Rest.

Try to turn to the right once more with your left hand leading the way, and note if the arc of the twisting movement is larger but nonetheless more comfortable.

The eyes are not only for seeing

Note the important role the eyes play in coordinating the musculature of the body; it is greater even than that of the neck muscles. Most parts of the body have two functions: the mouth serves for eating and speaking, the nose for smelling and breathing. The inner ear is instrumental in balancing the body in both slow and rapid movement in addition to its role in hearing. Similarly, the muscles of the eyes and the neck have a decisive influence on the manner in which the neck muscles contract. It is sufficient to recall climbing up or down stairs when the eyes did not see the floor at the end of the stairs to realize how great a part the eyes play in directing the muscles of the body.

Each eye separately, and both together

Sit down; bend your right leg to the right and draw your left leg toward your body. Turn your body to the left and lean on your left hand, placed as far to the left as possible within the limits of comfort. Raise your right arm to eye level and move it to the left on a horizontal plane. Look at your right hand and turn your head and eyes to any point on the wall, far to the left of your hand. Then look at your hand, then at the wall, then at your hand, repeating the movement about twenty times: ten with the left eye shut, and the movement from hand to wall executed by the right eye only; and ten with the left eye only. Then try to carry out the entire movement once again with both eyes open, to see if the range of the twisting movement to the left has increased. The improvement is often astonishing.

Bend your left leg backward, draw the right leg inward, and try to improve the movement to the right as well. Remember to carry out the exercise with each eye alternately open and shut.

Coordination of the eyes leads to improvement of the trunk

Rest. Observe which parts of your body are closer to the ground. This has been caused by your awareness of the eye movements. If the trunk stiffens again at some future time, it will be possible to note a corresponding lessening in the suppleness of the eye movements. It is possible to master the technique of coordinating eye movements in such a way as to improve the movement of the entire trunk.

Turn to the right; look to the left

Sit; bend your left leg backward and draw your right leg close to your body. Turn trunk, head, and shoulders as far to the right as is comfortable. Lean on your right hand, placed behind you. Lift your left hand, with the elbow bent, to eye level and move it to the right. Look at the hand and then to the left of it, at a particular point on the wall, and back to the hand, and continue twenty-five times. At each look you will see a little farther to the left.

Close one eye and carry out about ten such movements. Close the other eye and do the same. Make sure to keep your head still as you close each eye. Open your eyes and make another five movements. Remember the imaginary gentle upward tug at the top of your head. Afterward, try a simple movement to the right and see whether the arc you trace is wider and more comfortable.

Turn to the left; look to the right

Sit; bend your right leg backward, draw your left leg in, and turn trunk, head, and shoulders to the left as you lean on your left hand. Lift your right arm leftward at eye level. Look to the right of your hand many times. Close first one eye and then the other. Then open both eyes and make five movements with both eyes open. Observe the quality of the twisting movement as before. Lie on your back and rest.

Movement of the shoulder girdle to the right [Ill. 14]

Sit; bend your left leg backward and draw the right leg toward your body. Turn the entire trunk to the right. First lean on your right hand and then on your left as well, as they rest on the floor at some distance from each other. Lift your head and move your shoulder girdle to the right in such a way that the right shoulder moves backward and to the right and the left shoulder forward and to the right. Make sure that each of the shoulders moves decisively in its direction, the one backward and the other forward, until pressure is distributed equally over both hands.

As the shoulders move to the right, the head and eyes turn to the right as well as a matter of habit. Try to turn your head to the left as your shoulders move to the right, and to the right as your shoulders move to the left.

Observe your chest and your breathing, and continue to move your head in the direction opposite to that of your shoulders until the movement feels pleasant.

Transition from opposed movement to coordinated movement and back again

Continue with these movements of head and shoulders in opposite directions, but as you do so, without stopping, shift to coordinated movements, in which the head accompanies the shoulders both to the right and to the left. Then, without stopping as you move, resume the movement in opposite directions.

Stop and try to discover if there has been any improvement in the twisting and the feel of the movement. Lie on your back and examine the changes in the way your back touches the floor.

Movement of shoulder girdle to the left

Sit; move your feet to the right and carry out the entire exercise the opposite way: Move the head alternately in the same direction as the shoulders and in the opposite direction as in the preceding exercise. Remember, from time to time, to try to avoid trying to succeed.

Greater effort does not make better action

If you try to reach the limit of your abilities every moment, you end up with little more than aching muscles and straining joints. When you strain for results, you make it impossible to achieve even a part of the improvement that can be obtained through the breakdown of habitual patterns of movement and behavior, which is the aim of these exercises.

Improved differentiation of the movements of various parts of the body and of the relation between them leads to a lessening of the tonus (the degree of contraction caused by the involuntary centers) and a real increase in conscious control.

From time to time you should shake yourself out of your routine and ask yourself whether you are really doing what you think you are doing. Many people delude themselves into thinking that, because they sense an effort and wish their shoulders to move, their shoulders are indeed moving relative both to the floor and to their bodies, as they should.

Make sure that all the muscular effort is transformed into movement, for effort that is completely converted into movement improves both one's ability and one's body. Effort that does not turn into movement, but causes shortening and stiffening, leads not only to a loss of energy, but to a situation in which the loss of energy causes damage to the body structure.

Bend or incline head from side to side with body twisted to the right, then to the left

Sit; bend your left leg backward and bring the right one close to the body. Turn the whole trunk to the right and lean on your right arm. Increase the twist to the right a little and shift the right hand still farther to the right, so that the twist will cause only slight strain. Put your left hand on the top of your head and use it to help your head to bend to the right and left, so that the right ear will approach the right shoulder, and then the left ear approach the left shoulder. Be careful not to turn the head instead of bending it—the nose should continue to point to the initial frontal position even when the right ear is approaching the right shoulder and when the left ear is approaching the left shoulder.

Then bend the right leg backward and bring the left leg close to the body; turn the body to the left and lean on your left hand. Repeat the head bending movements with your right hand on the top of your head. You will be able to bend your head farther to the right and left if you help with a movement of the spine, which will bend to the left as your head goes to the right, and vice versa.

Swinging movements of the trunk, sitting

Sit on the floor and move both feet over to the right. Swing your trunk from right to left in light movements that slowly increase in size. Let both your arms be carried along by the movement of the trunk, precisely as you did in the standing position at the beginning of the lesson. Breathe freely in order to make the swinging movement easier.

After a few swinging movements reverse the movements of the head and eyes with respect to the trunk and arm movements so that the head and eyes will now move to the left while the trunk moves to the right, and vice versa. Without stopping the movement let the head again follow the trunk, and then reverse to the opposite movements.

Continue this alternate movement of the trunk until the changes from one to the other are smooth and simple. Carry out about twenty-five movements of each kind and then rest.

Repeat this exercise sitting in the opposite direction, with both legs turned to the left. Rest.

Sit up and observe the change in the quality and extent of the twisting movement since the beginning of the lesson.

Twisting of trunk in a standing position, with alternately rising heels

Stand up. Place your feet apart about the width of your pelvis and swing arms and trunk from right to left, the head moving with the body. As you move to the right, let your left heel rise from the ground; as you move to left, let your right heel come up. Make sure that the arm movement is free, and continue until you have carried out twenty to thirty swings from right to left.

When the head movements have become smooth and pleasant,

change their direction. Continue to turn the head in the direction opposite to that of the movement of the trunk until this also becomes smooth and easy. Reverse the direction again and move the head together with the shoulders. Try to change direction without interrupting the movement of the trunk.

Walk about and observe the changes that have taken place in the way you hold yourself erect and in your movements and breathing.

Lesson 11

Becoming Aware of Parts of Which We are not Conscious with the Help of Those of Which We are Conscious

There are parts of every body and every personality of which the individual is fully aware and with which he is familiar. For instance, almost everyone is ordinarily more conscious of his lips and fingertips than of the back of his head or his armpits. A self-image complete and uniform with respect to all parts of the body—all sensations, feelings, and thoughts—is an ideal which has been difficult to achieve up to now in man's state of ignorance. This lesson suggests techniques for completion of the self-image by comparing the sensation in parts of the body of which one is conscious with those parts of which one is not conscious. This experience helps you become aware of those parts that remain outside the range of active and conscious use in normal life.

An imaginary finger presses on your calf

Lie on your stomach. Stretch your legs in such a way that they are comfortably separated symmetrically to the spine. Place your hands one on top of the other on the ground in front of your head. Rest your forehead on the top hand.

Imagine that someone is pressing his finger on the heel of your right foot and draws it up the back of your calf from heel to knee. The pressure must make one feel the hardness of the leg bones;

the imagined finger must not slip right or left. Therefore one must stretch out the foot and the toes while the heel continues to point upward.

A ball rolls on the buttocks

Now try to imagine an iron ball rolling along your leg, from the middle of the heel to the knee and back again. The ball will follow the path of least resistance—the path that was chosen by the imaginary finger—so that it deviates neither to the right nor to the left. Try to identify in your mind all the points along its path, to make sure that the ball will not skip any of them.

Think of the pressure of the finger and then of the iron ball until you have found all the points you are not sure about. This needs no movement. Go on imagining the ball as it rolls from the knee toward the thigh and onto the large buttock muscle, the gluteus.

Find the thigh bone; start at the knee and move the ball toward the buttock. When you approach the buttock, you are less sure which direction to follow. Try to find where the ball would roll if you lifted your leg. Go on rolling the ball, back to the knee and thence to the heel, and then back to the buttock until all the points on its route are clear to you.

The ball on the back of your left hand

Stretch your left arm forward, comfortably bent at the elbow, and imagine the same heavy iron ball resting on the back of your hand.

Find the spot where the ball could rest without falling. Try to roll it toward the elbow; imagine the exact, firm course along which it would roll to the elbow and back again. Then imagine the same line of movement with someone running his finger along it, and go on doing this until it is entirely clear to you.

Continue in the same way from the elbow to the shoulder, and clearly note the course of the ball and of the finger. Return them slowly to the back of your hand, and from the back of your hand to your shoulder and the shoulder blade. Here, too, the final path of the ball is not clear.

Return to the right leg

Return to the right leg. Try to raise your heel and your calf a little, and imagine the points of contact along the path of the ball as it rolls up the back of your leg. Let the ball go on rolling slowly from the knee to the thigh, and see where it rolls when it reaches the buttock.

Note the muscular mobilization in the left shoulder as the ball rolls along its path.

From right thigh to left shoulder and back

Try to imagine the ball as it continues rolling on its path—from the knee, along the thigh, onto the pelvis, and toward the left shoulder blade. Find the exact point at which the ball crosses the pelvis in order to get to the waist and from there, along the spine, to the left shoulder blade.

Raise the shoulder blade slightly and let the ball roll back along the same course—to the spine, the waist, the pelvis, and the right thigh. As you do so, find the point at which it crosses the buttock on its way to the knee and the heel. Trace this line clearly, precisely, and continuously.

From the back of the left hand to the right heel and back

Return the ball to the back of the left hand. Lift the hand slightly so that the ball rolls down to the wrist; lift it a little higher, so that the ball rolls as far as the elbow, and still farther, till it reaches the shoulder blade. To keep the ball rolling, one must organize the body so that the point ahead of the ball along its course is lower than the ball, or that the point on which the ball rests is slightly higher than the point ahead.

Roll the ball from the shoulder blade along the spine, the buttock, and the thigh to the heel.

Raise your right leg slightly and let the ball roll as far as the buttock and then along the spine. Continue to move your body in such a way that the ball will roll to the shoulder blade, the shoulder, the elbow, and the forearm, as far as the back of the hand. To do this the arm must be stretched in such a way as to allow the ball to roll along a path free of sharp turns, so that it won't fall.

Go on alternately raising your arm and your leg, making sure that the ball's movement along its course is perfectly clear to you, that it moves at a regular pace, and that you know where it is at every moment.

The ball rolls in a groove

Place your left ear on the floor, straighten your left arm slightly at the elbow, and raise your body in such a way that the ball will be able to roll, as within a groove, from hand to heel and back again.

Note the course that the ball takes, and make sure that you have a clear notion of where to roll it.

Curve the body

Lift your left arm and right leg and balance your body in a slightly arched position, without straining. Roll the ball to and fro in the lumbar curve with rapid, light movements, so that it rolls a little toward the arm and a little toward the leg. Note the ball at every point, and try to determine what you are doing to make it roll in each direction.

Continue rolling the ball in the lumbar curve. Raise your arm and leg with light movements, leaving your left ear turned toward the floor. Gradually increase the scope of the movement so that the distance the ball travels increases each time, until it travels all the way from hand to heel with every oscillation.

Stand up slowly and walk about in the room. Notice whether

you feel anything out of the ordinary in your left arm and right leg, and along the path of the ball in general.

From left heel to right hand and back

Lie on your stomach again. Spread your legs apart and stretch your right arm over your head. Lay your right ear on the floor. Place the ball on the heel of your left foot and roll it to the knee and back to the heel; and again from the heel, along the same line, along the spinal column to the right shoulder blade; then from the shoulder blade to the elbow and along the forearm to the back of the hand—and back to the heel.

Note whether, at first, you think differently about this arm and leg than you did about the earlier pair. Think about the ball and its path, as you did before, until you can locate the ball at any moment and till you have a clear, precise idea of its pathway.

Move the ball at an even pace

When the path of the ball is really clear, the arm and the leg tend to lift themselves to return the ball to the heel and the back of the hand. Let them rise with a small, slow, and very light movement; otherwise the ball will stray off course. Try to move in such a way that the ball travels at an even pace throughout its course. Note that you must activate each part of the body at a different moment in order to allow the ball to continue moving toward its destination. You must direct the ball to the spot you are thinking of; otherwise the ball will not know where to roll.

The ball in the small of the back, with a rocking motion

Place the ball in the small of the back. Lift your arm and your leg slightly and rock the ball with small movements alternately toward the arm and the leg. Gradually increase the amplitude of the rocking movements so that the ball finally travels from the back of the hand to the heel with each movement.

Stand up and walk a little. Observe whether the feeling is different from the last time you got up and whether you can define the changes that have taken place in the back and within the body. Where do you feel different than you did before?

From the nape to the coccyx and back

Lie on your stomach. Spread your legs and arms with your hands stretched upward, over your head. Place your chin (not nose) on the floor. Place the ball on the back of your neck, between the shoulders and the head. Lift your head a little and gradually try to move the ball with a slow head movement down in between the shoulder blades. You will have to organize the shoulders, chest, and back in such a way that the ball finds a convenient place to roll in. Carry it downward from that spot, with a slow movement. To do this you must raise the breastbone so that the ball can roll down the back along that part of it corresponding to the chest until it reaches the pelvis, making sure that it does not slip in either direction.

Move the ball back toward the head. You must raise the buttocks and organize the stomach, the back, and the shoulders so that the ball can roll onto the nape; the nape itself must be lowered so that the ball can roll onto it. The knees remain on the floor throughout.

Roll the ball down to the pelvis and then back to the nape, each time carrying out the necessary movements more slowly and more clearly. Make sure that the head does not lean sideways.

With legs lifted

Spread your legs and this time lift them slightly off the floor; roll the ball from the head to the pelvis and back again without lowering the legs.

Lower the legs and continue as before. Observe the difference between the two kinds of movements.

With right leg and left arm raised

Return the ball to the small of the back. Raise the right leg and the left arm and roll the ball, with light movements, to the back of the hand, and then, by way of the spinal column, to the heel. Gradually increase the amplitude of the movement to end in a bold swing.

With right hand and left leg raised

Raise the right hand and left leg and proceed as above. Think primarily of the course the ball takes to be able to locate it and direct it wherever you wish.

Return the ball to the middle of the pelvis and roll it toward the nape and back again to the pelvis.

Test your imagination

Lie on your back, stretch your arms to the sides, spread your legs, and imagine patterns of movement for the ball that will enable you to sense your image in the front of the body with clarity equal to that with which you sensed your back after the preceding exercises.

Lesson 12
Thinking and Breathing

Some methods use improvement of breathing as the key to the improvement of personality. We change our breathing when we hesitate, become interested, startled, afraid, doubtful, make an effort, or try to do something. Our breathing is affected in different ways, from our completely holding our breath to shallow and rapid breathing that seems like an inability "to get any air."

Most people do not use the increased vitality that can be obtained from full and regular breathing, in accordance with man's nervous and physical structure; in most cases they do not even know what such breathing means.

In this lesson you will try a form of breathing that you can easily convert into habit to improve your general ability.

Absorbing more oxygen means greater vitality

Every living cell absorbs oxygen and rejects it again in the form of carbon dioxide. If the cells of the human brain are cut off from fresh oxygen for as little as ten seconds, the body dies or suffers serious harm.

A healthy lung is capable of inhaling more than a gallon of air, but it cannot expel the last remaining pint, even with a conscious effort. Under average conditions, when an individual is not hurrying or making any special physical effort, he does not use all his breathing apparatus, and at each breath he inhales and expels only about a pint of air. As such partial breathing is sufficient in a state of rest, it is easy to see that a slight increase in breathing—to perhaps as much as one quart at each breath —will improve all oxidation processes and general metabolism.

The desired improvement cannot be obtained by speeding up the breathing process, for quick breathing does not allow enough time for the air to be warmed up sufficiently before it reaches the lungs. The best way to improve breathing is to use the entire breathing apparatus, if only partially, but more than in the minimum breathing process that is carried out sluggishly.

Structure of the lungs

There are two lungs, the right and the left. The right one is very much larger than the left, being both longer and wider, for the left lung must share space in the chest with the heart and a large part of the stomach. The difference in size between the two lobes is so great that the bronchi have three branches on the right side and only two on the left.

Below the lungs is a muscular structure something like a vaulted sheath. This is the diaphragm, which is linked to the third and fourth lumbar vertebrae by two powerful muscles. (There are no muscles in the lungs themselves. The muscles with which we breathe are the upper muscles in the chest, linked to the nape, the rib muscles, and the muscles of the diaphragm.)

The lungs are more like a viscous liquid than a solid, for they expand into any empty space with which they are in contact. They are enveloped by a strong membrane connected with the walls of the chest, whose movements cause the lungs to change in volume as air is inhaled and exhaled.

The respiratory system

Our breathing system is complicated. We breathe in different ways when we are asleep, running, singing, or swimming. The only thing all forms of breathing have in common is that when we inhale air enters the lungs and when we exhale it is expelled, because the entire system is so constructed as to increase the volume of the lungs for breathing in, and to reduce it for breathing out.

This increase in volume can be produced by a movement of the chest in front, behind, or at the sides, or by an up and down movement of the diaphragm. In general, only a part of this system is used, and that not to its fullest extent. All the possible forms of breathing are used simultaneously when breathing must be speeded up, as after rapid and prolonged running.

The diaphragm

When the muscles of the diaphragm contract, the sheath is drawn down toward the lumbar vertebrae and the curvature reduced. The lobes of the lung are also drawn downward; their volume increases and air is inhaled. When the muscles relax the elasticity of the stretched tissues draws the diaphragm back again and the air is expelled. The muscles of the ribs and chest also play their part in this movement, of course. As we exhale the curvature of the diaphragm is increased and it becomes vaulted. As we breathe in, the curvature is reduced and it is pulled down.

The chest

As we breathe in the breastbone moves forward and upward. The ribs also perform a double movement similar to that of the breastbone. The muscles that cause the breathing movement in the upper part of the chest also pull the neck vertebrae forward. The movement of the lower ribs, the so-called floating ribs, which are not connected to the breastbone, is more effective in causing the volume of the lungs to expand than that of the upper ribs located just beneath the collarbone. In the upper part of the chest—where the lungs are narrow and flat and the movement of the ribs constricted—a large muscular effort causes only a relatively small increase in the volume of the lungs. The floating ribs, on the other hand, move much more freely: the ribs move out farther with a relatively small muscular effort and expand the lungs in their widest section.

Coordination of chest and diaphragm in normal and paradoxical breathing

When the chest widens to allow us to inhale, the diaphragm drops and flattens out and helps to increase the volume of the lungs. As we exhale, the chest is contracted and the diaphragm regains its curvature upward. There is also a paradoxical form of breathing in which the diaphragm operates in the opposite way, and some individuals always breathe this way. Most animals that roar or low use paradoxical breathing; that is, they increase the volume of their stomach when they breathe out and by this means produce a loud sound. In the Far East it is customary to cultivate paradoxical breathing, for it is considered to give better control over the limbs and a more erect posture than ordinary breathing.

In fact, we use paradoxical breathing whenever we must make a sudden violent effort, even if we are not aware of it. It is therefore important to learn something about it.

The lung: a passive organ

Expansion of the chest causes the lungs to be sucked outward by their covering membranes and the air that enters the lung flattens it out against the walls of the chest. When the muscles that have expanded the chest relax we begin to expel the air, a process helped by the weight of the lung and the elasticity of the connective tissues. As the air is expelled, the lung recedes from the inner walls of the chest and shrinks. It is, of course, also possible to reduce the volume of the lungs actively by deliberately expelling the air inside it.

Breathing and posture

Air must penetrate through the nose and mouth into the windpipe, bronchi, and lungs—and be expelled again—properly, in order to supply sufficient oxygen at all times and under all conditions throughout a person's life. If breathing is internally disrupted we cannot survive more than a few seconds, though we can hold our breath for a few minutes. Most of the muscles of the respiratory system are connected to the cervical and lumbar vertebrae and breathing therefore affects the stability and posture of the spine, while conversely the position of the spine will affect the quality and speed of breathing. Good breathing therefore also means good posture, just as good posture means good breathing.

Breathing in the area of the right shoulder

Lie on your back. Draw up your knees so that your feet can stand on the floor, close your eyes, and try to remember the movements of the lung and diaphragm as they were just described. Breathe slowly, in small, short steps, making many movements of the chest and abdomen for every time you inhale or exhale. Observe your chest in your imagination, and see in your mind's eye how it pulls your right shoulder, between collarbone and shoulder blade, every time air is drawn into this section. Observe this spot only as you breathe and skip in your imagination the expelling half cycle. Air reaches this point from the middle of the body, about halfway between the breastbone and the floor, where the bronchi are, three on the right and two on the left. The chest sucks the lung in various directions at once: to the right shoulder, between the collarbone and the shoulder blade (in the direction of the ear), to below the armpit, to the shoulder blade resting on the floor, and to the front of the chest.

As it takes some time to visualize all these details, you may take several partial breaths as you think out the sequence. Observe the pulling action of the muscles that take part in the movement.

Passage of air to the right upper bronchi

Now imagine the passage of the air as it enters your nostrils and goes to the back of your palate and into your windpipe. Think only about this point every time you breathe in, until all these parts are known and familiar to you. When this first section has become clear, follow the air in its passage from there to the right upper bronchi. Now go back to the nostrils; when these are familiar move on to the palate, all down the windpipe, to the space around the windpipe, to the air that flattens the lung against the walls of the chest, and is itself forced upward, down toward the floor, toward the shoulder and the armpit.

Passage of air to the right lower bronchi

Now imagine the path of the air entering the nostrils and flowing past the palate to the windpipe and into the third, lower bronchi, through which air reaches the lower part of the right lobe of the lung where it borders on the liver. Observe this path only with every breath.

As you observe this path, keep in mind the space around this third lower bronchus, the direction in which the air presses around the liver and against the hips: forward, downward, toward your legs, and to the sides.

The two right bronchi

Now with each breath follow the path of the air through the nostrils, past the palate, to the windpipe, and through both bronchi, upper and lower. Imagine the right lobe of the lung expanding. Its upper part moves up and its lower part down at the same time, so that the whole right side is stretched and the distance between the pelvis and the armpit is increased.

With every breath think how the air is filling the space at the top and the space at the bottom and how the right lobe is being stretched by the diaphragm. Observe whether you feel anything in the lumbar vertebrae as you do this. The third and fourth hip vertebrae should rise from the floor as the two muscles of the diaphragm pull the lung downward.

The middle bronchus

Now imagine the middle bronchus on the right. Try to think of the passage of the air all the way from the nostrils, past the palate, and into the center bronchus. The stretching of the right lobe upward and downward has in any case already stretched it in the middle as well. Now, in addition to this expansion, the lobe will also be widened forward and backward; that is, it will become thicker in relationship to the floor. Think of the inner parts of the lung, and of how the chest is "sucking" it in all these directions.

Repeat the whole process

Try to repeat the whole exercise of the breathing in half cycles of spreading and widening from beginning to end, and note which sections you can feel clearly and which you cannot feel at all. Repeat this until the whole process is continuous and fully familiar. Then think about the shrinking of the right lung as you breathe out. The air now moves back from the top of the shoulder, from the shoulder blade and the chest, returns through the bronchi to the windpipe, past the palate, and comes out through the nose. As you breathe out the air is squeezed from the lung as from a sponge.

Lower and middle sections

Imagine the same action in the lower and middle parts of the right lung. Observe how the lung moves back from the diaphragm and the ribs, from the direction of the floor, and from the breastbone and forces out the air. Breathe slowly, in the ordinary way, so that you can identify the entry of the air, the lengthening of the right side, the expelling of the air, and the contraction of the side. Get up and observe the difference you can now feel between the right and the left side.

Let the right lung slide

Sit on the floor with your legs crossed. Close your eyes, bend your head forward, clasp your hands, and place them across the back of your head, letting your elbows hang down loosely between your knees. If you find it difficult to bend over like this, you will also discover that at the point where the spine is not flexible the lung does not move and does not breathe; what is difficult to enact is also difficult to imagine. In this sitting position again think of the passage of air through the nostrils and past the palate into the windpipe; watch the stretching of the right lung to the shoulder blade at the top and down past the liver, and also through the middle bronchus. See whether in this position you can think that you feel the lung slide inside past the whole length of the lining of the lung. Note at which points in your thinking the lung does not slide freely. When you have identified these points and can imagine them easily, your head will bend forward farther and more easily.

Get up, walk about, and observe the marked difference you can feel in your breathing on the right and left sides.

You will agree that it is difficult to believe that thinking about the movement of the air through the windpipe and the bronchi has really directed it to the points in your right lung only. Perhaps the muscles of the side you were thinking about began to work a little differently after you had been practicing for a few minutes so that your breathing in and out on that side was also changed somewhat. In any case, the muscles on the right side of the chest and diaphragm worked the same as on the left side during every breath you took, for it is very difficult to learn to move one side of your chest without letting the other side follow it. The difference that you feel derives from nothing but the changes in the working and organization of the muscles produced by your simultaneous attention to their working and the spatial orientation of the parts of your body that you were watching.

These changes have, in fact, taken place in the upper part of your nervous system and not in the muscles themselves, and cover the whole right side. You will therefore be able to observe a corresponding difference in your face, and the right arm and leg will feel longer and lighter. If you look in a mirror you will see that the feeling is not imaginary, for the right eye will really be opened wider, and the folds in the right side of your face less pronounced than in the left.

Parallel movements on the left side

Sit on the floor, cross your legs, and this time think about the stretching of the left lung. The head slowly begins to rise with each breath. Observe how the breath spreads all along the spine with the movements of the head. At the points where the spine is stiff and the chest does not move and does not suck the lung after it sufficiently, it does not slide. Continue until you can think that it does. See whether you can identify the movement of the diaphragm pulling the lumbar vertebrae.

Get up, move about, and note the difference you can feel after you have made much of the breathing process conscious.

Breathing with the left lung, with head tilted right

Sit on the floor again. Bend your right leg back, bring your left foot close to you, lean on the floor with your left hand, and tilt your head so that your right ear approaches your right shoulder. Remain in this position and fill your left lung with air. In your imagination stretch it on the left side, up into your shoulder in the direction of the ear and downward at same time. In this way the lung will slide to fill up the entire space on the left side of the chest. Breathe out and imagine the withdrawal of the lung in the whole chest. Note your head, which will no longer be sunk down onto the shoulder. The inability to bend your head farther stems from lack of flexibility in the chest, whose muscles are still too greatly contracted. Breathing is incomplete in any part of the chest that is not fully flexible.

Breathing with the right lung

Sit on the floor and breathe as before. Imagine the lengthening of the right lung and then its withdrawal from the walls of the chest when you breathe out and the feeling of shrinking, as though it were literally being pulled away. Note that when you observe what is happening on the right side, the head and whole trunk lean to the left when you are in the lengthening stage and return to the middle when you breathe out.

Stand up and check the changes that you can feel in your body.

Postscript

Contemporary research into the behavior of animals in their natural habitat has produced increasing evidence that the elements of social structure are not man-made in the sense that music and mathematics are man-made. The close link to a particular home or territory, loyalty to herd or flock, hostility to members of a neighboring herd, and even the fixed hierarchy within the herd all indicate that territorial wars and struggles for power and position derive from mankind's animal ancestry and are by no means man's own invention. The aggressive impulse has always been the stumbling block in the way of man's attempts to improve himself. The few exceptional men who really sought peace and true brotherly love reached this condition by perfecting their awareness, not by suppressing their passions.

If it is really true that instincts come to us as a matter of inheritance, just as awareness is inherited, then it will be preferable to perfect our awareness rather than to suppress the animal that is in us. Awareness is the highest stage in man's development, and when it is complete it maintains a harmonious "rule" over the body's activities. When an individual is strong, so are his passions, and his ability and vitality are on the same scale. It is impossible to suppress these prime movers without reducing his total potential. The improvement of awareness is preferable to any attempt to overcome instinctive drives. For the more nearly complete a man's awareness becomes, the more he will be able to satisfy his passions without infringing on the supremacy of awareness. And every action will have become more human.

In the present century the younger generations have liberated themselves from the conventions of their predecessors in the fields of morals, sex, and aesthetics. Only in a few areas such as science and the creation of material goods can these generations continue in the footsteps of their elders without doing violence to their own feelings. In these two fields they tread the established road; in all other aspects of life they are either in open rebellion or simple confusion.

Increase of awareness will help them to find a way out of confusion and free their energies for creative work.